Positive Options for
Polycystic Ovary Syndrome

About the Authors

Christine Craggs-Hinton is the mother of three children. She had a career in government until 1991, when she developed fibromyalgia, a chronic-pain condition. She took up writing for therapeutic reasons and has since written *Living with Fibromyalgia*, *The Fibromyalgia Healing Diet*, and *The Chronic Fatigue Healing Diet* (all published by Sheldon Press, London). She writes for the Fibromyalgia Association UK and the related *FaMily Magazine*, and she also writes fiction.

Adam Balen, M.D., is a consultant in reproductive medicine and surgery at Leeds General Infirmary, where he participates in the management of an in vitro fertilization unit. The author of five books, including *The Practical Management of Polycystic Ovary Syndrome*, he has also written numerous articles and chapters on a variety of topics related to reproductive medicine for journals and edited collections. He has had a particular interest in the causes and management of polycystic ovary syndrome for many years.

Dedication

WE WOULD LIKE TO DEDICATE THIS BOOK TO ALL WOMEN WITH PCOS. MAY YOU SOON FIND YOURSELVES WITH FEWER SYMPTOMS AND ENJOYING LIFE TO ITS FULLEST.

Other titles in the Positive Options series

Positive Options for Antiphospholipid Syndrome (APS) by Triona Holden

Positive Options for Crohn's Disease by Joan Gomez, M.D.

Positive Options for Hiatus Hernia by Tom Smith, M.D.

Positive Options for Living with Your Ostomy by Dr. Craig A. White

Positive Options for Seasonal Affective Disorder by Fiona Marshall and Peter Cheevers

Forthcoming

Positive Options for Reflex Sympathetic Dystrophy (RSD) by Elena Juris

Positive Options for Colorectal Cancer by Carol Ann Larson

Ordering

Trade bookstores in the U.S. and Canada please contact:

Publishers Group West
1700 Fourth Street, Berkeley CA 94710
Phone: (800) 788-3123   Fax: (510) 528-3444

Hunter House books are available at bulk discounts for textbook course adoptions; to qualifying community, health-care, and government organizations; and for special promotions and fund-raising. For details please contact:

Special Sales Department
Hunter House Inc., PO Box 2914, Alameda CA 94501-0914
Phone: (510) 865-5282   Fax: (510) 865-4295
E-mail: sales@hunterhouse.com

Individuals can order our books from most bookstores, by calling (800) 266-5592, or from our website at *www.hunterhouse.com*

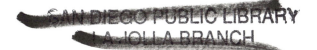
Positive Options

for

Polycystic Ovary Syndrome

Self-Help and Treatment

Christine Craggs-Hinton and
Adam Balen, M.D.

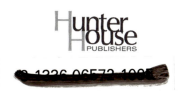
Hunter House
PUBLISHERS

Hunter House Inc., Publishers
PO Box 2914
Alameda CA 94501-0914

Library of Congress Cataloging-in-Publication Data

Craggs-Hinton, Christine.
[Coping with polycystic ovary syndrome]
Positive options for polycystic ovary syndrome : self-help and treatment / Christine Craggs-Hinton and Adam Balen.— 1st ed.
p. cm.
Includes index.
ISBN 0-89793-437-7 (pbk.)
1. Stein-Leventhal syndrome—Popular works. I. Balen, Adam H. II. Title.
RG480.S7C73 2004
618.1'1—dc22   2004002783

Project Credits

Cover Design: Brian Dittmar Graphic Design
Book Production: Hunter House
Copy Editor: Kelley Blewster
Proofreader: John David Marion
Indexer: Nancy D. Peterson
Acquisitions Editor: Jeanne Brondino
Editor: Alexandra Mummery
Publicist : Lisa E. Lee
Foreign Rights Assistant: Elisabeth Wohofsky
Customer Service Manager: Christina Sverdrup
Order Fulfillment: Washul Lakdhon
Administrator: Theresa Nelson
Computer Support: Peter Eichelberger
Publisher: Kiran S. Rana

Printed and Bound by Bang Printing, Brainerd, Minnesota

Manufactured in the United States of America

9 8 7 6 5 4 3 2 1   First Edition   04 05 06 07 08

Contents

List of Figures

Author's Note

This book was written by Christine Craggs-Hinton. Invaluable input into the scientific and medical chapters was contributed by Adam Balen, M.B., B.S., M.D., FRCOG, consultant obstetrician and gynecologist and specialist in reproductive medicine and surgery, and medical advisor for Verity, a support group for people with polycystic ovary syndrome. Adam Balen has also checked and approved the full content of this book.

Important Note

The material in this book is intended to provide a review of information regarding polycystic ovary syndrome. Every effort has been made to provide accurate and dependable information. The contents of this book have been compiled through professional research and in consultation with medical professionals. However, health-care professionals have differing opinions, and advances in medical and scientific research are made very quickly, so some of the information may become outdated.

Therefore, the publisher, authors, and editors, as well as the professionals quoted in the book, cannot be held responsible for any error, omission, or dated material. The authors and publisher assume no responsibility for any outcome of applying the information in this book in a program of self-care or under the care of a licensed practitioner. If you have questions concerning your health, or about the application of the information described in this book, consult a qualified health-care professional.

Introduction

Polycystic ovary syndrome (PCOS) is a common condition, yet many doctors are not sufficiently enlightened about it to be able to make a diagnosis readily. It seems that this unfortunate fact is often compounded by women failing to describe all their symptoms to their doctor. It is easy to understand why this is the case, given that women with PCOS are likely to experience such seemingly unrelated problems as facial hair, acne, and irregular periods, none of which are the easiest things to talk about.

The symptoms of this complex condition are caused by a hormonal imbalance. There are a variety of approaches to treatment, and they may differ over time depending on the needs of the individual patient. Practitioners of orthodox medicine frequently advise taking the contraceptive pill and perhaps other hormone preparations, which can work to great effect and are discussed in this book. However, these therapies do not provide a cure. Fortunately, great improvements may also be made by using more natural methods, and this book attempts to discuss all of these therapies, from diet and lifestyle changes to advice on how to improve your self-image, how to get the most from your relationships, and how to reduce stress.

Chapter 1

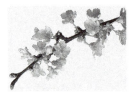

What Is Polycystic Ovary Syndrome?

Polycystic ovary syndrome, known as PCOS, is the most common endocrine (hormonal) disorder in women of reproductive age. It is characterized by a collection of symptoms, which include the following:

- excessive facial and/or body hair (hirsutism)
- weight gain
- adult acne or excessively oily skin
- absent or irregular periods
- difficulty getting pregnant
- hair loss (alopecia)

Other symptoms that may be associated with PCOS include the following:

- mood swings
- tender breasts
- miscarriage
- bloating

◆ fatigue

◆ joint pain

◆ depression

◆ pelvic or abdominal pain

In addition, women with PCOS are at greater risk of developing some longer-term health problems. These include the following:

◆ late-onset (type-2) diabetes

◆ high cholesterol levels, heart disease, and stroke

◆ cancer of the lining of the uterus (endometrium)

The main problems experienced by women with PCOS are menstrual-cycle disturbances (irregular or absent periods), difficulty controlling body weight, and skin problems (acne and unwanted hair growth on the face or body). Not all women with PCOS experience all of these symptoms, and a woman's problems may change over time. In particular, if a person with PCOS becomes overweight, her problems will generally worsen.

Polycystic means "many cysts," and a *syndrome* indicates a collection of more than one symptom. About 30 percent of all women have multiple cysts on their ovaries, although only a smaller percentage will develop the symptoms associated with PCOS. Not all of the above symptoms need necessarily occur together to lead to a diagnosis of PCOS.

PCOS was first described by Irving Stein and Michael Leventhal in 1935.[1] In fact, until fairly recently it was known as *Stein-Leventhal syndrome*. Because it was impossible in the 1930s to carry out the blood tests and ultrasound scans that we take for granted today, a diagnosis at that time was based on absent periods, hirsutism, and obesity. The combination of these three symptoms is now seen as the classic feature of PCOS. However, it is clear that the syndrome comes with a wide spectrum of possible symptoms, a fact that can make diagnosis difficult.

Various studies have shown certain symptom patterns in women with PCOS. As you can see from Table 1, irregular periods appear to be the most common symptom, closely followed by hirsutism, infertility, and being overweight.

Table 1: Frequency of symptoms in women with PCOS

Symptom	Percentage of PCOS patients with the symptom
Irregular periods (oligomenorrhea)	60–90
Excessive facial or body hair (hirsutism)	70–80
Infertility	40–60
Being overweight (obesity)	30–50
Absence of periods (amenorrhea)	30–50
Acne	20–35

If one looks at the statistics in another way, about 80–90 percent of women with irregular periods have PCOS, about 90 percent of women with acne have PCOS, and about 95 percent of women with hirsutism have PCOS.

Let's take a closer look at several of these symptoms.

Irregular or Absent Periods

A "regular" menstrual cycle is defined as being between 23 and 35 days from the start of one period to the start of the next; in addition, a "regular" cycle does not vary by more than two days from its average length. If your menstrual cycle, from the day you start one period to the day you start your next period, varies by more than two days it can be classified as irregular. Similarly, it is irregular if your periods occur closer together than 23 days, or farther apart than 35 days.

Having a cycle longer than 35 days is known as *oligomenorrhea* (infrequent menses), whereas going six months or more without a period is known as *amenorrhea* (absent menses). In women with oligomenorrhea, ovulation (the release of an egg from the ovary) either may be irregular or may fail to take place at all. This situation can be controlled by the use of the contraceptive pill, which is of most benefit to women who require a reliable form of contraception. Preparations of the hormone progesterone may also be used to help to regulate the menstrual cycle. (See Chapter 3 for a discussion of medications that help to regulate menstruation.) In some cases, irregular or absent periods may also be controlled by more natural means, which are outlined in Chapters 5 and 6.

Hirsutism

The embarrassing condition known as *hirsutism* is defined as excessive facial or body hair, or both. The distribution commonly occurs in a male pattern; the possible areas affected include the upper lip, chin, upper and lower back, chest, upper and lower abdomen, upper arm, thighs, and buttocks.

The problem can be treated by the use of chemical depilatory creams, bleaching, laser, electrolysis, waxing, and shaving. If you do not want to become pregnant, your doctor may prescribe a contraceptive pill (such as Yasmin) to reduce the growth of unwanted hair. Since this type of therapy can take many months to show benefits, the hair-removal techniques mentioned above may be used in the meantime. (See Chapter 3 for more details on the medications that treat hirsutism and Chapter 5 for further information on hair-removal techniques.)

Infertility

Fertility depends on many factors. For a start, ovulation—the release of an egg from the ovary—must occur; the male partner's sperm need to function normally; and the sperm require a normal passage to reach the Fallopian tubes, where fertilization takes place. It is a fact, though, that fertility declines with increasing age—particularly the age of the female partner. Fertility testing is usually started after a couple has been trying to get pregnant for a year, since by then it is expected that about 85 percent of young couples (those under the age of 30) should have conceived. If there is an obvious reason for reduced fertility (for example, infrequent menstrual periods and therefore few ovulations), it is reasonable to start tests and treatment right away.

The irregular ovulation often seen in PCOS is the most common reason for difficulty in getting pregnant. A woman normally releases an egg once a month and can conceive at this time. When the number of times she ovulates is reduced, the number of times she can become pregnant is also reduced. However, several medications exist that can effectively kick start the ovaries into action, and they are discussed in Chapters 3 and 4.

Sadly, women with PCOS appear to have a tendency to miscarry. Recurrent miscarriage (that is, three or more miscarriages) has been linked with PCOS. The exact cause is often unknown but may be related to hormonal disturbances and being overweight. Weight loss in overweight women with PCOS can dramatically improve their chances of getting pregnant and carrying the pregnancy to term.

The normal function of the ovaries and how the ovaries are affected by PCOS are described in detail in Chapter 2.

Weight Gain/Being Overweight

Weight-management problems are common in PCOS. Some sufferers put on extra pounds starting in puberty, when the female sex hormones can first go awry because of PCOS. In most cases, a normal body mass index (BMI) is between 20 and 25, but women with PCOS often have a higher BMI. BMI is calculated by dividing one's weight in kilograms by the square of one's height in meters. To determine your weight in kilograms, divide your weight in pounds by 2.2046. To determine your height in meters, divide your height in inches by 39.37. Therefore, a person weighing 140 pounds and with a height of five feet, five inches—or 65 inches—would calculate her BMI as follows:

Step 1 140 pounds ÷ 2.2046 = 63.5 kilograms

Step 2 65 inches ÷ 39.37 = 1.65 meters

Step 3 1.65 x 1.65 = 2.7225 (square of height in meters)

Step 4 63.5 ÷ 2.7225 = 23.32 BMI

Unfortunately, weight gain can be a double-edged sword in PCOS. Women with polycystic ovaries who would not normally develop the syndrome sometimes start having symptoms when they become overweight. And since a woman with PCOS may have a slower metabolism than normal, weight loss can be hard to achieve.

Although some women with PCOS experience no particular pattern of fat distribution, many others put on weight around their middle. Consequently, the ratio of the measurement around the waist to the measurement around the hips often increases. This is commonly known as being "apple-shaped" (as opposed to "pear-shaped").

Being overweight worsens the symptoms of PCOS—especially acne, unwanted hair, and infertility. Weight reduction will generally improve control of the menstrual cycle, reduce the heaviness of the menstrual flow, and improve fertility and the other symptoms of PCOS. A healthy eating plan combined with aerobic exercise is the only real answer for weight loss (for more information about diet and exercise, see Chapter 5). However, some drug therapies may also help (see Chapter 3). If you want to lose weight, try to enlist the support not only of your doctor, but also of your family and friends. Ask to be referred to a dietician if you feel you are unable to follow the diet recommendations in this book.

Acne

Acne is common in teenagers. However, when it persists into adult life (beyond the age of 20), the most common cause is PCOS. Acne and excessively oily skin are largely a result of the increased testosterone levels brought on by PCOS. Testosterone causes the sebaceous glands, which lubricate the skin, to go into overdrive and produce relatively large amounts of oil. The excess oil clogs the skin's pores (the tiny tunnels leading to the skin's surface). Bacteria exist on the surface of everyone's skin, but when the pores become blocked, the bacteria multiply within the sebaceous gland, causing pimples and small cysts to appear. Acne can appear on the chest and back as well as on the face.

Over-the-counter creams and lotions may be of some benefit in treating acne, as may the long-term use of certain antibiotics (erythromycin and tetracyclines—although tetracyclines must not be taken if you are trying to get pregnant). However, these products will not treat the underlying hormone imbalance that causes the acne in the first place. Again, if you do not wish to get pregnant, your doctor may prescribe a contraceptive pill, some of which offer the additional benefit of acne reduction.

Some women report a worsening of their acne when they discontinue taking the contraceptive pill. Whether you use the pill or not, the best long-term treatment for acne is probably an improved diet (see Chapter 5) and drinking lots of water. Some people find regular use of tea tree oil or hemp oil effective. These oils are applied directly to the skin. (For more information on the medications used to treat acne, see Chapter 3.)

Dealing with Embarrassing Symptoms

Women with PCOS can find themselves having to deal with a whole host of embarrassing symptoms. It is one thing to visit your doctor because you feel under the weather, and another to visit your doctor because you have hairy nipples and facial hair. Most women believe that a tendency toward excess facial or body hair is something they were born with. They are surprised to learn that this condition can be a symptom of hormonal disturbances and may therefore be treatable. It is the same with persistent adult acne. Women tend to think acne is "just one of those things"—

that they have drawn the short straw where zits are concerned and that they just have to come to terms with the problem.

Furthermore, who wants to see the doctor because they've been putting on weight? If they're not laughed out of the doctor's office, many believe, surely they'll simply be told to stop eating so much. Being overweight can be embarrassing, not least because onlookers may jump to the conclusion that you have been overeating—in other words, indulging yourself.

Frequently, when women tell their doctors that their periods are irregular, the problem is treated in isolation. This is generally because women don't even think to mention unwanted hair, acne, and an increase in weight; what can these other problems possibly have to do with irregular periods? It is a fact, though, that the doctor needs to see the whole picture before he or she can make a correct diagnosis. The doctor cannot know just by looking at you that you wouldn't be caught dead without your weekly application of a depilatory cream.

In the same way, your doctor will have no way of knowing that you've tried every diet ever promoted, but to no avail. It is also possible, if the doctor gives you only a cursory glance, that he or she won't realize you have acne beneath all that concealing makeup. As we said earlier, PCOS is not the easiest condition for either the patient or the doctor to recognize.

In many cases, the doctor may consider the symptoms of hair loss, weight gain, fatigue, irritability, and irregular periods as indicators of stress, for stress is known to have wide-ranging effects. Alternatively, mood swings, fatigue, pelvic and abdominal pain, and irregular periods may be attributed to premenstrual syndrome (PMS). When suffering from a condition that is as difficult to diagnose as PCOS, the patient herself may have to do some of the groundwork and then bring the condition to her doctor's attention. In the end, the responsibility for our own health lies with us—not with our doctors.

A Condition to Be Taken Seriously

To continue on the subject of embarrassing symptoms, some women are even reluctant to inform the doctor that their periods are irregular. Many of us were brought up thinking of our menstrual period as "the curse." We believe that it naturally causes moodiness, pelvic and abdominal pain, and even acne. Those with scanty periods may see the doctor, only to be told they should consider themselves lucky because a light flow is far easier to deal with than a heavier one. But long gaps between periods can lead to abnormal thickening of the uterine lining, which, in turn, can increase the risk of endometrial cancer. It is therefore essential to ensure that the lining of the uterus is shed at least once every three months to prevent abnormal thickening. Scanty or irregular periods are not always a symptom of PCOS, but they usually are.

The trouble with PCOS is that if it is left untreated, the long-term health risks mentioned at the beginning of the chapter may eventually rear their ugly heads. These health risks are discussed in more detail in Chapter 2.

Infertility is another, shorter-term side effect experienced by some sufferers of PCOS. Women tend to expect to have little or no trouble getting pregnant and so generally put off trying to conceive until the time is right—after all, pregnancy and childbirth are usually considered the most "natural" female functions of all. However, when there is no sign of a pregnancy after months or even years of trying…well, it can feel like the end of the world. Infertility problems can cause great heartache. There are solutions, however, so keep reading.

What Does It Feel Like to Suffer from PCOS?

Although the symptoms of PCOS vary a great deal from person to person, sufferers often complain of feeling tired. They are likely to be concerned about their periods; as noted above, the periods are either heavy and frequent, scant and infrequent, or nonexistent.

Consequently, sufferers of PCOS may worry about their ability to have children. Excessive facial or body hair, acne, and weight gain often arise in puberty, but women can develop these symptoms in their 20s, 30s, and even 40s. Also, because many of the symptoms rate high on the embarrassment scale, the affected woman will doubtless find her confidence shaken. It can be frightening to develop such symptoms seemingly out of the blue.

When hair loss from the head is a problem as well as hair growth in a male pattern on the face and body, some women secretly fear they are turning into men. To believe that your femininity is being threatened can be nothing less than terrifying. It doesn't even take hair loss or hirsutism for some women to feel they are losing their femininity; putting on weight and developing acne can have the same effect. Obviously, this state of affairs can lead to psychological problems. The emotional aspects of PCOS are discussed in Chapter 7.

The fact that some doctors may at first find nothing wrong or may attribute the symptoms to stress doesn't help matters. When a correct diagnosis is finally achieved, the patient may experience feelings of relief mixed with fear about what may lie ahead. However, please be assured that medications, lifestyle adjustments, and stress-management techniques can make an enormous difference in PCOS.

Can the Cysts Linked to PCOS Be Removed?

It is a misconception that ovarian cysts are the cause of PCOS. They are, in fact, a result of the hormonal disturbances within the ovary. In PCOS the ovarian follicles fail to develop normally, and ovulation fails to occur on a regular basis. This is why in PCOS patients the little follicles or cysts remain in the ovary and can be clearly seen on an ultrasound scan. The cysts themselves are very small (only 0.08–0.3 inches in diameter); they usually cluster in groups of 10 or so around the ovary's perimeter. Removal of the cysts doesn't cure the condition, because doing so doesn't resolve the hormonal imbalance. In fact, if the cysts are removed, more will form in their place.

Note that what are generally referred to as *ovarian cysts* are different from the cysts that develop with PCOS. Ovarian cysts usually occur by themselves and can grow to a much greater size (as large as an inch or more). A woman with PCOS has as much of a chance as a woman with normal ovaries of developing a very large ovarian cyst. If this occurs, it may require surgical removal.

Is PCOS Curable?

Although PCOS is a malfunction of the body that cannot be permanently "cured," it should not be regarded as a disease. The symptoms can be controlled with medical treatments combined with the right lifestyle changes and, perhaps, complementary therapies. As a result, your life can become far more productive, in every sense of the word. Instead of telling yourself you have an incurable condition, try to think of it as an ongoing health concern requiring long-term treatment. You've taken an important step by reading this book, as the goal of this book is to help you develop a treatment plan that is right for you.

Chapter 2

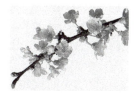

What Causes Polycystic Ovary Syndrome?

P COS is a complex disorder in which the function of the ovaries is affected and the body's metabolism may be disturbed. A condition known as *insulin resistance* is also likely to be present.

Many factors can apparently predispose a woman to PCOS, including familial (genetic) links, environmental factors, lifestyle factors (for example, diet, which affects body weight), and imbalances in the production of hormones from the various glands (the ovaries, the adrenal glands, the pancreas, and the pituitary). Lifestyle and environmental factors can also play a role in either triggering or worsening the condition (see Chapter 5).

The cause and course of the condition have been examined in some well-documented studies.[2,3]

A Familial Link

By investigating large families, researchers have found that PCOS has a genetic component. Specifically, different aspects of the syndrome can be inherited by different family members as a result of faulty genes.[4] There may be male-pattern baldness (where the hairline recedes at the front and on the crown) in male family members, and polycystic ovaries in their female relatives. As a result of studies such as these, experts believe that consideration of a woman's relatives can determine whether or not she will suffer from polycystic ovaries.

Of course, because ultrasound scanning was not readily available before the 1980s, there was no way for a woman to know for sure whether or not her relatives had polycystic ovaries (or polycystic ovary syndrome), even though the symptoms are quite easy to define. Still, it is possible to follow the trail of the disorder through the generations, because certain illnesses—the long-term health risks of PCOS—may be seen in older relatives. These include conditions that occur in both sexes (adult-onset diabetes, high blood pressure, and being overweight) as well as those that occur only in female family members (infertility, hirsutism, menstrual problems, and endometrial cancer).

It is not yet fully understood why one woman with polycystic ovaries has a regular monthly cycle and normal hormone levels, while another develops PCOS, but it is thought that genetic factors play a role. Each cell in the body has 23 pairs of chromosomes (making 46 chromosomes altogether, including an X and a Y chromosome in men and two X chromosomes in women). Each chromosome contains thousands of genes, each of which controls the production of the proteins that tell the body how to grow and function. Many diseases and medical conditions, including PCOS, occur because of faults in this genetic messenger system. Often a combination of genetic abnormalities is present, which is why different combinations of symptoms can manifest themselves in different people.

Research suggests that more than one gene is involved in causing PCOS. A 1997 study showed that, in PCOS, one of the faulty genes is involved in the first stage of testosterone production, which accounts for the raised levels of this hormone in a PCOS patient's bloodstream.[5] Experts believe that this gene probably interacts with other genes and with the environment to produce the final clinical picture. In another study, it was discovered that there is also a link between a specific variation in the insulin gene and the failure to ovulate in women with PCOS.[6] Research into the genetics of PCOS continues.

It is interesting that there also appear to be ethnic variations in the development of PCOS. There is a higher incidence of PCOS among women from southern Asia than in white Caucasian women. The reason for this difference remains unknown.

Normal Ovarian Function

In PCOS, the hormonal household is in total disarray. However, in order to explain the many malfunctions, we first need to understand how the normal ovary works.

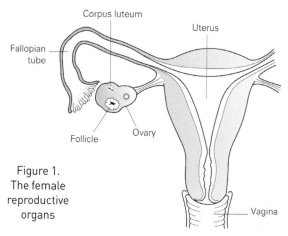

Figure 1.
The female
reproductive
organs

The ovaries are a pair of almond-shaped organs located deep within the female pelvis, behind the uterus and Fallopian tubes (see Figure 1). The number of eggs that the ovaries carry is allotted before birth, when the ovaries are first formed. This means that no new eggs are produced, and the eggs that a woman ovulates at the age of 40 are 40 years old. It appears that the better eggs are ovulated earlier in a woman's life, and also that the eggs carry an increased risk of genetic or chromosomal abnormalities as they grow older. This helps to explain the decline in fertility and the increased risk of miscarriage as women grow older, as well as the increased risk of chromosomal defects in children born to older mothers—Down's syndrome is just one example.

A girl's eggs lie dormant until she reaches puberty. At the start of puberty, a substance called *gonadotrophin releasing hormone* (GnRH) is released by the hypothalamus (the body's hormonal control center, located near the base of the brain) and secreted into the nearby pituitary gland. The pituitary is the command center for the release of hormones from other glands, such as the ovaries, adrenal glands, and thyroid. GnRH triggers the release of *luteinizing hormone* (LH) and *follicle-stimulating hormone* (FSH), which travel to the ovaries. As a result, the hypothalamus–pituitary–ovary pathway is fully awakened, and the girl will start her menstrual periods (see Figure 2).

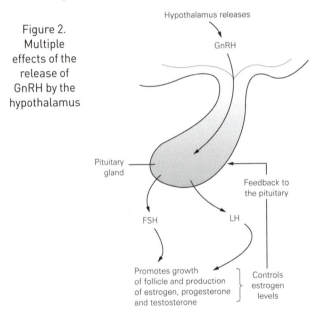

Figure 2. Multiple effects of the release of GnRH by the hypothalamus

Hypothalamus releases

GnRH

Pituitary gland

Feedback to the pituitary

FSH

LH

Promotes growth of follicle and production of estrogen, progesterone and testosterone

Controls estrogen levels

The normal menstrual cycle is often considered to be 28 days in length, but in reality it can range from 23 to 35 days, as discussed in Chapter 1. What is important is the regularity of the cycle, which should not vary by more than one or two days (plus or minus) from the individual woman's average cycle length. The control of the cycle is determined by the release of GnRH from the hypothalamus and by feedback from the ovaries in the form of hormonal messages to the pituitary and hypothalamus. Stress and a change in body weight can upset the release of GnRH and disturb the monthly cycle.

The first half of the cycle—the two weeks before the egg is released from the ovarian follicle—is known as the *follicular phase*. It is this "growing" phase of the cycle that varies between women, whereas the second half of the cycle, known as the *luteal phase*, is usually fairly constant in length (14 days for most women). The luteal phase occurs after the egg has been released and, generally, picked up into the Fallopian tube (ovulation). The follicle that has released the egg changes into a *corpus luteum* in the second half of the cycle, and it is this structure that produces *progesterone* after ovulation. Progesterone plays an important role in preparing the endometrium (uterine lining) for the implantation of an embryo. An embryo results when an egg is fertilized by a male sperm. Under normal circumstances, the embryo should implant in the endometrium and ultimately develop into a baby.

The Follicular Phase

During the follicular phase, follicle-stimulating hormone (FSH) is released from the pituitary gland. FSH, as its name implies, stimulates the follicles in the ovary to develop their eggs. One follicle in particular will quickly become dominant and will thus become the most likely to produce a mature egg. As soon as this occurs, the other eggs will stop ripening, allowing the dominant follicle to grow to a size of about 0.8 inches. At the same time, luteinizing hormone (LH) is released from the pituitary, and, together with FSH, the production of the hormones estrogen and testosterone are promoted. Estrogen production increases as the follicle continues to grow. It is normal for the ovary to also produce testosterone, because estrogen cannot be made without the presence of testosterone.

In the middle of the menstrual cycle, there is a final surge of LH. This causes the follicle to rupture and the egg to be released into one of the Fallopian tubes, from where it is transported toward the uterus. Ovulation predictor kits, which are available in most drugstores, rely on the measurement of LH in the urine to detect the timing of ovulation.

The Luteal Phase

During the luteal phase of the cycle, the follicle changes in function to form the corpus luteum. The corpus luteum produces progesterone, the dominant hormone for the remaining two weeks of the cycle. Progesterone ensures that if fertilization has occurred, the thickened womb lining will secrete the nutrients that will feed the egg.

If fertilization occurs as the egg travels down the Fallopian tube, the egg continues to the uterus, where it is implanted in the uterine lining. After implantation, the placenta of the developing pregnancy produces a hormone called *human chorionic gonadotrophin* (hCG)—the hormone that measures positive in a pregnancy test. This hormone stimulates the corpus luteum to continue to produce progesterone until about 12 weeks into the pregnancy. The embryo immediately begins to divide repeatedly until a fetus develops. The placenta secretes hormones for the duration of the pregnancy.

If fertilization does not take place, production of progesterone and estrogen ceases, and the collapsed follicle (corpus luteum) begins to shrivel. The thickened uterine lining then starts to break down and is shed as a menstrual period. The whole process of the menstrual cycle recommences at this point.

Abnormal Ovarian Function in PCOS

In PCOS, it appears that a malfunction within the hypothalamus–pituitary axis causes abnormal levels of hormones to be released. Levels of LH are often elevated, and it is the combination of this hormone and insulin that stimulates the production of testosterone by the ovaries. All women produce testosterone, which in normal circumstances is converted into estrogen as the follicle grows, but in women with PCOS, testosterone levels are higher than normal.

If an ovarian follicle fails to grow to maturity, as is often the case in PCOS, then the testosterone finds its way into the body's circulation and may have effects on the skin, resulting in acne, hair loss, and unwanted hair growth. Testosterone may also be converted into estrogen in the fat stores of the body, causing the woman to put on weight.

Estrogen is required by the endometrium (uterine lining) in order to help it to develop. Unfortunately, the abnormally high estrogen levels resulting from PCOS increase the thickening of the womb lining, so that eventually it may break down of its own accord, causing either a period or else spotting and bleeding between periods.

The peppering of partially developed follicles around the periphery of the ovaries are the cysts that can be seen on ultrasound scans. Because of abnormal hormone levels, they have failed to develop into normal egg-producing follicles. However, even when a woman's cycle is irregular, a normal ovulation may occur from time to time, albeit in an unpredictable manner. Irregular cycles and problems with ovulation are the reasons why some women with PCOS experience difficulty getting pregnant.

High Levels of LH

As stated above, in the middle of the menstrual cycle, a final surge of LH is required to complete the development of the egg and allow it to be released from the follicle. However, when levels of LH are high throughout the cycle, as is often the case in PCOS, the development of the oocyte (egg cell) within the follicle may fail to take place properly. It is thought that if ovulation occurs in the presence of a constantly high LH concentration throughout the follicular phase of the cycle, a time lapse between the ripening of the egg and its release may cause it to be prematurely aged—meaning either that it cannot be fertilized—or may result in an abnormal fertilized embryo. The ultimate rejection of such an embryo by the body gives us a possible explanation for the occasional miscarriages seen in PCOS patients.

Increased Levels of Testosterone

When the ovaries themselves fail to work as they should, their core and outer coating become thickened—and it is this thickened material that produces higher amounts than are desirable of testosterone and other hormones that we normally associate with men (these hormones are known collectively as *androgens*). Testosterone is present in both sexes, but men produce 10 times more than women. As mentioned earlier, excess production of testosterone in women is the cause of many PCOS symptoms, such as acne, excessive facial and body hair, and the failure to ovulate (anovulation). Elevated testosterone levels is the most common hormonal abnormality in PCOS, but not all sufferers are affected. On the other hand, some women are seriously affected.

It may be helpful to appreciate that the normal blood testosterone level in women is 0.5–3.5 nmol (nanomols) per liter; in men it is usually 15–30 nmol per liter. Women with PCOS usually have a testosterone level of 2.5–5.0 nmol per liter. If the testosterone level is greater than 5 nmol per liter, it is important to look for other problems, such as testosterone-secreting tumors in the ovary or adrenal glands (which are very rare) and an uncommon condition called *congenital adrenal hyperplasia.*

Testosterone is carried in the bloodstream by a protein called *sex hormone–binding globulin* (SHBG). High insulin levels can suppress the production of SHBG so that the amount of active (or "unbound") testosterone is elevated, which is why some women can have quite profound signs of testosterone excess in the presence of a normal blood concentration of the hormone. This is particularly the case in overweight women with high insulin levels.

The mild elevations of testosterone levels seen in women with PCOS can cause distressing symptoms (acne, hirsutism, and thinning of head hair), collectively known as *androgenization* or *hyperandrogenism.* However, testosterone levels in PCOS never get high enough to cause "virilization," which can cause the voice to become deeper, the breasts to shrink, and the clitoris to enlarge. If these effects occur, it is necessary to seek expert medical advice because the problem is not being caused by PCOS.

Insulin Problems

In recent years it has become clear that there may be problems with insulin levels in cases of PCOS; in fact, an increased insulin level in the blood appears to be one of the causes of the condition, whether the woman is slim or overweight.[7] Insulin is a hormone that is normally released from the pancreas after a meal. It allows the cells of the body to take up energy in the form of glucose, from which glycogen is released. Glucose is also stored in the liver as glycogen. Glycogen is a type of glucose that acts as a storage molecule and is used as a backup source of energy when normal glucose levels have fallen. It is vital that glucose in the body is maintained at a stable level, because brain function and normal body metabolism depend on it.

When glucose levels are inadequately controlled, diabetes is the inevitable result. High levels of blood glucose (hyperglycemia) can cause excessive thirst, frequent urination, and, ultimately, fainting and coma. Low levels of blood glucose (hypoglycemia) can cause shakiness, dizziness, hunger, headaches, moodiness, and confusion. If we eat more carbohydrate (which is converted to glucose) in one meal than can be stored by the liver and the muscles, the excess is converted to fat and stored in the fat cells.

Studies have found that PCOS patients have difficulty converting glucose to energy—a condition called *insulin resistance*. In an effort to compensate, the pancreas produces more insulin, which creates higher circulating levels of insulin than normal—a situation called *hyperinsulinemia*. The result is often abnormal cholesterol and lipid levels, weight gain, irregular periods, higher levels of androgens (the male hormones that all females have in low levels), infertility due to disturbance of ovulation, and an increased likelihood of developing diabetes.

The excess insulin not only stimulates higher than normal secretion of androgens from the ovaries, but also it appears to affect the normal development of the ovarian follicles. Because the incidence of diabetes in overweight women with PCOS is 11 percent, long-term screening of patients is advisable.[8] Metformin, a diabetes treatment known as an insulin-sensitizing agent, can lower blood-sugar levels and reduce high insulin levels. Weight reduction may also achieve the same effect. (See Chapter 3 for more information on metformin.)

One study found insulin resistance in 30 percent of slim women with PCOS and in 75 percent of overweight women with PCOS.[9] The study also reported a far higher percentage of women with a raised testosterone level in the latter group. This explains why overweight women with PCOS are more likely to suffer from hirsutism and infertility than slim women with PCOS.

Women with PCOS who have high levels of circulating insulin due to insulin resistance are at increased risk of developing diabetes during pregnancy, a condition known as *gestational diabetes*. Gestational diabetes can usually be managed by dietary modification. However, it sometimes requires drug therapy (including insulin injections). It is therefore recommended that overweight women lose weight before getting pregnant. Gestational diabetes generally disappears after pregnancy, but it signals an increased risk for the development of diabetes again in later life.

Women who do not take steps to control their diabetes before they conceive run an increased risk of miscarriage and of difficulties during pregnancy and childbirth. They also have an increased risk of giving birth to babies with congenital malformations.

PCOS and Being Overweight

Being overweight may dramatically increase insulin levels and exaggerate all of the symptoms of PCOS. Estrogen is made in the fat tissues and can lead to overgrowth of the endometrium. If ovulation is not occurring and the endometrium becomes progressively thickened, the menstrual period, when it finally arrives, can be very heavy and painful. Furthermore, if there are excessively long gaps between periods, or if the periods are not happening at all, there is the risk of developing an abnormally thickened endometrium and, rarely, cancer of the uterus. To prevent these things from happening, it is important to have a period once every three months, at the very least.

Losing weight not only can reduce the symptoms of PCOS, but also it can normalize ovulation and thereby boost fertility. In a study of overweight women with PCOS who were not ovulating, 82 percent began to ovulate after losing weight. In a different study, all but one woman with PCOS and fertility problems went on to conceive after losing weight. Yet another study examining the relationship between being overweight and fertility problems in PCOS found that once women lose weight, many of their hormonal problems are resolved.

Weight loss can be difficult, but it will result in lower insulin levels, which in turn reduces testosterone production by the ovaries. It can be challenging to sustain a healthy eating regime, and it is unfortunately quite common for women with PCOS to get into bad habits and develop disordered eating patterns, such as binge-eating and self-induced vomiting (known as *bulimia nervosa*). Indeed, it has been suggested that nearly two-thirds of women with bulimia also have PCOS. If you have this kind of problem, see the Resources section (located in the back of the book) for the names of organizations that offer help with eating disorders. It is important that bulimia be tackled correctly and sensitively to prevent further problems from arising.

The Long-Term Health Risks of PCOS

The long-term health risks of PCOS are mainly related to the insulin problems and raised testosterone levels that generally play a part in the condition. High levels of insulin are associated with an increased risk of developing type-2 diabetes. Type-2 diabetes generally requires strict diet control or possibly drug therapy. Between 25 and 35 percent of overweight women with PCOS show signs of type-2 diabetes by their 30s; the condition becomes even more common in women in their 40s and beyond. To prevent the onset of diabetes, it is recommended that you follow a healthy eating plan and exercise regularly (see Chapter 5).

The hormone changes characteristic of PCOS increase the chance of later developing high blood pressure and high cholesterol levels, both of which can lead to a greater risk of heart disease. Again, a healthy eating plan and regular exercise can greatly reduce these risks.

As mentioned previously, irregular or infrequent periods over a long period of time can lead to an increased risk of cancer of the endometrium (uterine lining). This risk is due to high levels of estrogen, which overstimulate the endometrium, causing it to continue to thicken. Normal shedding of the endometrium by way of regular periods effectively prevents endometrial cancer. If the endometrium appears thick on an ultrasound scan or if irregular, prolonged bleeding occurs, a biopsy of the endometrium may be recommended. This can be done in an outpatient clinic or as a day-stay surgical procedure. The uterine lining is first inspected by a fine scope (a hysteroscope), and then a curettage or endometrial biopsy is performed.

For women with no periods at all, use of a low-dose contraceptive pill can regulate periods and help avoid the risk of endometrial cancer. For those who cannot take the pill, progesterone hormone treatment can offer the same benefits. As long as a menstrual period occurs at least once every three months, the risks of developing endometrial cancer are minimal.

As stated previously, irregular and heavy periods can occur as a result of problems with ovulation. While it would seem that restarting ovulation is the best treatment, this is generally reserved for times when a pregnancy is desired. Ovarian-stimulation drugs have potentially troublesome side effects and need to be carefully monitored; thus, their long-term use is inappropriate. However, the contraceptive pill and progesterone hormone treatment can stimulate menstruation without ovulation.

There does not appear to be a link between ovarian cancer and PCOS.

Chapter 3

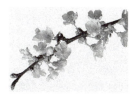

Getting Help from Your Doctor

If you think you have PCOS, it is important to secure a diagnosis as early as possible. Without treatment of some kind—either through conventional medicine or by following a holistic approach—long-term health problems become a greater risk. Treatment appears to be effective in the majority of cases, and early diagnosis has the benefit of improving your long-term health outlook.

Preparing to See Your Doctor

If you are reading this book, you probably either suspect you have PCOS or already have a diagnosis of PCOS. For those who suspect, we suggest that you write down all of your symptoms, even if some of them appear unrelated to PCOS. You may be suffering from another condition entirely. An abnormality of the pituitary or adrenal glands—a tumor, for example—can cause symptoms similar to those of PCOS. Obviously, if a tumor is detected, immediate treatment is essential.

Note that teenagers who have been taking the contraceptive pill to control heavy periods may start displaying the symptoms of

PCOS only when they stop taking the pill, even if it's several years after you were first prescribed it. In such cases, the diagnosis may be delayed for many years. In reality, the symptoms for which the pill was prescribed may have been the early manifestations of PCOS; when the individual stops taking the pill, the symptoms are unmasked once again.

It is important to feel that you have the support of your doctor. If you are nervous about seeing your doctor on your own, it may be helpful to take a good friend or close family member with you to your appointment.

Consider making the following preparations for your visit to the doctor's office:

◆ Make a list of all the symptoms you have experienced in the past four weeks. In addition to the main symptoms we've discussed in some detail (excessive facial or body hair, weight gain, acne, hair loss, and, if it is relevant, difficulty getting pregnant), your symptoms may include fatigue, depression, painful joints, bloating, tender breasts, and mood swings. Write down a full and precise description of each symptom.

◆ If you are having periods, write down a description of your monthly cycle, including the heaviness of the bleeding, how many days you bleed, and the average number of days from the start of one period to the start of the next one. Mention any spotting that occurs between periods.

◆ If you are not having periods, make sure to write that down. Try to remember when your last period was and make a note of that, too.

◆ Jot down any questions you want to ask the doctor. Doing so will act as a memory prompt when you're visiting with the doctor. It will also show the doctor that you feel the problem is serious.

At the Doctor's Office

Following these pointers should help you to get the best result from your doctor visit:

- Be as calm and relaxed as possible when talking to your doctor. Many doctors admit to feeling defensive and being less open-minded if the patient is even a little belligerent. In the same way, appearing nervous can have the effect of making you seem unsure about your symptoms. Writing down everything beforehand should give you confidence.

- Speak clearly and slowly so that your doctor misses nothing.

- Tell your doctor that you have read about PCOS and suspect that you have the condition.

- Each time your doctor asks you a question, be sure you understand the question before replying.

- The doctor may request that you undergo some medical tests, which is the result you want. If the doctor doesn't mention tests, make the suggestion yourself. In the unlikely event that your doctor doesn't think tests are required, be sure to ask what other causes there might be for your symptoms. Remember that if you are unhappy with your doctor's conclusions you are entitled to a second opinion.

What Tests Am I Likely to Undergo?

PCOS can easily be diagnosed by blood tests and an ultrasound scan.

Blood Tests

Blood tests help to rule out similar conditions and can confirm a diagnosis of PCOS. If you are having periods, your doctor will probably schedule you for a blood test during the first three days of your menstrual period. If you are not having periods, blood can be taken at any time, but the test may need to be repeated.

Your blood will most likely be tested for the following:

- *Androgen levels (testosterone and androstenedione).* Although not all women with PCOS have increased levels of the androgen hormones, these abnormalities are very common in PCOS.

- *LH.* Recall from the last chapter that this hormone stimulates the ovary to produce testosterone. Again, although high levels of LH are often seen in PCOS, there are many exceptions. Normal LH levels should not rule out a diagnosis of PCOS. Testing for LH is best carried out during the first three days of a menstrual bleed. If periods are absent or infrequent, a random blood sample can be taken.

- *FSH.* This hormone is a good predictor of the fertility potential of the ovaries. Testing for FSH should be performed on days one through three of a menstrual bleed, but it can be done randomly in cases where periods are absent or irregular.

- *SHBG.* Levels of this hormone may be low in women with PCOS.

- Insulin. Blood levels of insulin are not usually measured, since the test is complicated and therefore only performed as part of research. However, insulin resistance can be determined by performing a glucose-tolerance test. The test is performed on an empty stomach after an overnight fast. The patient drinks a sugary drink; her blood is then taken immediately, and again after two hours. A glucose-tolerance test should be carried out if the woman is overweight (body mass index greater than 30). However, South Asian women with PCOS, for example, are more likely to develop insulin resistance at a lower body weight than is typical in female Caucasians. For this reason, a glucose-tolerance test may be advised in non-Caucasian women if the body mass index is more than 25.

♦ *Thyroid function.* Some of the symptoms of PCOS are similar to those of thyroid malfunction, making this test necessary as a part of the diagnostic procedure.

♦ *Prolactin levels.* Prolactin is a hormone that, when elevated, can be associated with irregular or absent periods; its levels should therefore be checked.

♦ *Full blood count.* This test will show whether you have adequate red blood cells. The role of red blood cells is to carry oxygen throughout your body. If you have an inadequate number of red blood cells, the result is often fatigue and anemia.

If blood tests suggest that you have PCOS, your physician may send you for an ultrasound scan.

Ultrasound Scan

Ultrasound scans are performed either at the office of a radiologist or in a hospital. For external scans of the lower abdomen, a full bladder makes the reading clearer. For this reason you may be asked to drink up to two quarts of water beforehand. A small amount of clear gel is placed on the lower abdomen, and the probe is moved around the skin's surface. Ultrasound waves are bounced off the ovaries to create a picture. A woman with PCOS will have ovaries that show many tiny cysts around the edge of the ovary in a "pearl necklace" effect. These are the partially developed eggs that were never released from the follicles into the Fallopian tubes.

Women undergoing an internal scan—which involves placing a small ultrasound probe just inside the vagina—do not need a full bladder. An internal scan gives a clearer view of the ovaries and pelvic organs and should not cause pain.

If the scan reveals that the endometrium is thicker than 15 mm (about 0.6 inches), a period may be induced by specific medication, usually a short course of progestogen tablets.

What Happens after the Diagnosis?

Once your doctor has concluded that your problem is indeed PCOS, there are several possible courses of action. Conventional medical treatment—that is, drug therapy—is generally the first step in treating the symptoms, but if you wish to attempt to tackle the underlying causes of the disorder, you could also try the holistic approach, as discussed in the next chapter. Most doctors are pleased to hear that the patient is making efforts to help herself, as an adjunct to drug therapy. However, the medications offered generally give more immediate results and may be used until holistic treatments take effect. For women who find holistic treatments difficult to maintain or for whom the effect is less than desired, medications may be the only effective way forward.

Because many of the drugs that treat the symptoms of PCOS prevent pregnancy, your doctor will, first of all, want to know whether you are trying to get pregnant. Some medications should be avoided while you are trying to conceive (for example, tetracyclines, spironolactone, flutamide, finasteride); reliable contraception will therefore be advised if you are taking any of these. Remember that even if you are not having periods you may ovulate without warning from time to time. If you wish to prevent a pregnancy you must *always* use reliable contraception, even if your periods are nonexistent or infrequent. (Women with infrequent periods and no wish to conceive sometimes get pregnant and fail to realize that they're pregnant until it is too late to have the pregnancy terminated.)

Try not to feel daunted by the large number of medications presented in this book—it means only that there is a great deal of help available. It also means that if one type of drug is unsuitable for whatever reason, there is generally an equally effective alternative.

Medications That Regulate Your Periods

If you wish to prevent a pregnancy, a low dose of the oral contraceptive pill can regulate your monthly menstrual cycle. Any combined oral contraceptive pill (a COCP, which combines estrogen and progesterone) can achieve this. All COCPs may elevate the SHBG levels and also suppress testosterone production by the ovaries, thereby improving the symptoms of hyperandrogenism (the mild elevations of testosterone seen in PCOS). Sometimes Yasmin is prescribed, because in addition to bringing the cycle to a normal 28 days and normalizing blood loss, it also contains progestogens, the hormones that help to counteract the effects of androgens (testosterone and others). Yasmin contains drospirenone, a derivative of spironolactone, which is the main antiandrogen used in the United States. An oral contraceptive sometimes prescribed to treat PCOS in the U.K. and other countries is Dianette, which contains cyproterone acetate, an antiandrogen that can help to combat acne and hirsutism. However, Dianette and cyproterone acetate are unavailable in the United States.

Unfortunately, the oral contraceptive is known to exacerbate the problem of insulin resistance; it is also linked to many other possible side effects. These include fluid retention, acne, weight gain, headaches, nausea, high blood pressure, and an increased risk of blood clots. If you have problems, you should talk them over with your doctor. There may be another contraceptive pill that will better suit you.

Many women report that the pill masks their PCOS symptoms while they are using it, but that when they stop taking it, their symptoms worsen. Indeed, this is precisely how the pill is designed to work. However, all drugs may have adverse effects, so it is generally a matter of weighing whether the benefits are worth the potential side effects. Each case is highly individual; some PCOS patients will benefit more from using the pill than will others.

An alternative to the COCP is one of the progestogen-only preparations, which can induce regular withdrawal bleeding if taken on a cyclical basis (for example for 12 days every one to three months to induce a bleed). Such preparations include medroxyprogesterone acetate (Provera). The side effects linked with these drugs are probably worse than those of the COCP; they include weight gain, fluid retention, abnormal production of breast milk, gastrointestinal upset, breast pain, and acne. Obviously, some of these possible effects, if they arise, are counterproductive to women with PCOS, and alternative medications may need to be explored. Because women with PCOS are thought to be at increased risk of later developing heart disease, a COCP that contains agents that reduce the effects of dietary fats could be used. Ask your doctor about such medications.

Any irregular bleeding while you are taking hormone-based medications should be reported to your doctor, who may advise an ultrasound scan or curettage surgery. And finally, all sexually active women should have a cervical (Pap) smear at least once every three years.

As an alternative to medications, a progestogen-releasing intrauterine coil or intrauterine device (for example, Mirena) may be offered. The IUD can effectively prevent the abnormal buildup of the endometrium (uterine lining). The main side effect may be unpredictable light bleeding or discharge, and periods may occasionally stop altogether. However, this is safe because it occurs when the endometrium has become thin.

Medications That Treat Hirsutism and Acne

Hirsutism and acne are the result of elevated levels of testosterone in the female body. Recall from Chapter 2 that testosterone levels are dictated by the amount of SHBG in the blood. High levels of insulin lower the production of SHBG from the liver and so increase the levels of active (free) testosterone.

Your doctor may use a standardized scoring system such as the modified Ferriman and Gallwey score to evaluate the degree of hirsutism before and during drug therapy. The Ferriman and Gallwey score enables a record to be kept of the amount of unwanted hair covering the different parts of the body. It is, of course, difficult to make such an assessment if methods such as shaving, waxing, electrolysis, or laser are being used to deal with the unwanted hair.

Besides oral contraceptives, spironolactone (Aldactone) is another option for treating stubborn acne and hirsutism; however, it frequently causes erratic periods and thus is often given with a low-dose contraceptive pill. Spironolactone is a mild diuretic; it reduces water retention and lowers blood pressure in those with elevated blood pressure. It is commonly used to treat PCOS when it is unsafe to use the contraceptive pill—for example, in cases of extreme obesity, in smokers over age 35, or in cases of high blood pressure.

Other medications aimed particularly at hirsutism include the antiandrogens flutamide and finasteride. As mentioned above, reliable contraception is essential with these drugs. Their side effects include tiredness, mood changes, and reduced sex drive. As with other antiandrogens, flutamide can impair liver function, so patients taking the drug should undergo blood tests every six months.

Owing to the slow rate of hair growth, all hirsutism treatments must be continued for up to 18 months before a response may be seen. During that time, depilatory creams, electrolysis, laser, bleaching, waxing, and shaving can be used to treat the problem.

Medications That Treat Obesity

Medications are now available that inhibit the absorption of fat from the diet. However, since they inhibit good fats as well as bad fats, they should be used only when all else has failed and only in the short term to start the process of weight reduction. There is no substitute for a healthy weight-loss plan. For more information on diet, see Chapter 5.

Medications That Treat Insulin Resistance

The first line of attack against insulin resistance is weight loss. The next step is to consider a drug called metformin (brand name Glucophage), an antidiabetic drug that is often used to treat non-insulin-dependent (or type-2) diabetes. For women with PCOS, metformin has been shown to lower levels of insulin, testosterone, and LH, and to raise levels of SHBG.[10] As a result, menstruation can often be regulated, ovulation may occur, and the symptoms of androgen excess (hirsutism, acne, etc.) may decline.[11]

In a 1998 study, metformin was shown to improve menstrual patterns in women suffering from PCOS, with minimal endocrine and metabolic effects.[12] As a bonus, when combined with a healthy diet and exercise, metformin can cause weight loss in those who are overweight. All in all, metformin offers benefits for both short-term and long-term health. Not all women lose weight while taking metformin, however, and again there is no substitute for a healthy diet and exercise. Note that metformin is not yet a licensed treatment for PCOS and can be prescribed for PCOS only by an endocrinologist or specialist in reproductive medicine. Metformin therapy may be continued in the long term, but as a precaution it should be stopped during pregnancy (although detrimental effects on either the mother or the fetus have not been reported).

When starting to take metformin, patients will often experience an upset stomach, diarrhea, and flatulence (gas). These problems usually resolve after the first week or two and can be minimized by taking the drug with a meal and by starting on a low dosage. It is recommended that patients start with one 500-mg pill daily for the first week and then during the second week increase to taking 500 mg twice a day. If stomach upsets are minimal after the second week, the dose can be raised to 850 mg twice daily. Other side effects linked with metformin include various endocrine disorders (hormonal problems), repeated infections, agitation, stress, allergic reaction, and skin rashes.

People taking metformin should discontinue the medication immediately if they experience shortness of breath, severe muscle weakness, or chest pain. It should also be stopped 48 hours before surgery and 48 hours before an X-ray study in which dye is administered (such as an intravenous pyelogram). It should not be taken by people who use alcohol excessively.

You will be asked to return to your doctor three months after starting metformin. If you have successfully ovulated and wish to conceive, therapy will continue for another three months to see if you can become pregnant. As stated, metformin should be stopped if pregnancy occurs.

Your doctor may wish to prescribe the insulin-lowering agents pioglitazone (brand name Actos) or rosiglitazone (brand name Avandia), or both, either in place of metformin or to work alongside it as a combination therapy. These medications have been known to reverse the endocrine abnormalities seen in PCOS within two or three months. They can result in diminished facial or body hair, regulation of the menstrual cycle, normalization of high blood pressure, decreased hair loss from the head, weight loss, and improvement in fertility. Some women have even conceived during their first ovulatory cycle after taking these medications. Studies have shown that by six months, over 90 percent of women treated with these medications may resume regular periods.

Women taking pioglitazone or rosiglitazone will be required to see their doctor every two months for monitoring of their liver function. Ovulation will be monitored and, after four months, laboratory tests reevaluated. The levels of C-peptide and of insulin secretion may also be tested. If therapy fails to prove successful, the dosage of drugs may be increased or combinations prescribed.

The few studies conducted into the use of insulin-sensitizing drugs as a treatment for PCOS suggest that they may well be beneficial. They appear to help regulate menstruation and facilitate ovulation. Some women experience an improvement in their weight and in their cholesterol levels. Weight reduction is a more variable finding. One study looking at ovulation in particular found that it occurred in 34 percent of the women who were taking metformin.[13] When metformin was combined with a drug called clomiphene citrate (brand name Clomid; see Chapter 4 for more information), 90 percent of women ovulated, whereas only 8 percent of those on only clomiphene citrate ovulated. These study groups were made up of overweight women with PCOS. Whether the same results would be seen in women of normal weight has not yet been established.

It is important to note that pioglitazone and rosiglitazone carry the same possible side effects as metformin. The side effects linked to clomiphene citrate include hot flushes, abdominal discomfort, blurred vision, and enlargement of the ovaries.

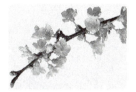

Chapter 4

Getting Pregnant

As we have seen, several types of medication are capable of kick starting normal ovarian function and may therefore help you to achieve a pregnancy. As well as detailing the most effective of these medications, this chapter discusses some of the medical procedures involved in fertility treatment. (See Chapter 7 for help with the emotional repercussions that may arise during this difficult time.)

Preparing to Get Pregnant

It is important to follow certain general health measures when trying to conceive. For starters, a healthy diet is essential (see Chapter 5). Smoking is not only harmful to your health; it also reduces your chances of having a successful pregnancy. It is therefore important not to smoke if you are trying to have a baby. In addition to reducing fertility, smoking is associated with an earlier onset of menopause and an increased risk of miscarriage, stillbirth, and sudden infant death syndrome (SIDS). It is also a good idea to abstain from alcohol, which is believed to have a significant effect on both female and male fertility.

You should also be aware that if you are trying to conceive, you should be taking 0.4 mg (400 micrograms) of folic acid daily. This has been shown to reduce the incidence of some developmental anomalies in the baby, such as spina bifida.

Weight Reduction in Overweight Women with PCOS

It is estimated that 85 percent of women with ovulatory difficulties suffer from PCOS. Because the syndrome is more common in overweight women, weight reduction should be a woman's first step toward increasing her chances of conceiving. Weight reduction may even trigger spontaneous ovulation. The necessary amount of weight loss is probably less than you think; a reduction of only 5 percent of a PCOS patient's current weight is associated with an increased number of ovulatory cycles. Furthermore, even if spontaneous ovulation does not occur, losing weight increases a woman's chances of responding to the drugs that promote ovulation. It is therefore sensible that you should immediately start following a healthy eating plan (see Chapter 5). Doing so will not only benefit your pregnancy and unborn child, but also it will also help to reduce the symptoms of your PCOS.

Initial Fertility Tests

If you have been diagnosed with PCOS and the time is right for you and your partner to start trying to start a family, you should go to your doctor right away and ask to be referred to a fertility specialist. First, however, your own doctor may initiate some tests.

Initial fertility tests include checking to make sure you are immune to rubella (German measles) before you conceive. Blood hormone levels (FSH, LH, testosterone, thyroid function, and prolactin) will be checked, usually during the first three days of your menstrual cycle, or at random if you do not have periods. Progesterone levels will be checked approximately seven days before your expected period (on day 21 of a 28-day cycle), although there is little point in measuring progesterone if your periods are very irregular. At some stage, your partner will probably be asked to provide a semen sample for analysis.

Checking Ovulation

Many women like to use home predictor kits to determine whether ovulation is occurring. It is our advice is that such tests are generally not worthwhile; they can be expensive and inaccurate if your cycle is erratic, and if your cycle is regular, then you *are* ovulating and there is no need to do your own tests. The sort of tests we are referring to most commonly measure LH in the urine. LH is the hormone that is released in a surge about 40 hours before ovulation takes place. Some women with PCOS have high circulating levels of LH throughout their cycle, causing the urine to test falsely positive when a surge is not actually happening.

Because the body's temperature rises by 0.4–0.9°F shortly after ovulation (an effect of progesterone), temperature testing used to be popular. However, because this method is less reliable and causes stress, it is no longer recommended.

When to Make Love

Couples wishing to conceive worry about when to make love. They often think it is best to delay having intercourse until around the time of ovulation. While it is, of course, true that sperm need to be present in the Fallopian tubes when the egg is released, it is actually not good for men who are trying for a baby to wait for long periods of time between ejaculations. This is because sperm, unlike eggs, is manufactured daily and stored before release—and the longer the sperm is stored, the older it gets. The sperm count may slowly increase, but sperm function tends to decline as the sperm ages.

The optimum time between ejaculations is two to three days, so it is advisable to try to make love at least every three days during the first half of the cycle and perhaps a little more frequently (every one to two days) around the time of anticipated ovulation. If you are having regular periods (that is, with a cycle length of between 23 and 35 days, but not varying by more than two to three days from its average length each month), then chances are you are ovulating 14 days before your period is due. Remember that it is the *second* half of the cycle, after ovulation, that is the most consistent in terms of length.

At the Fertility Clinic

When you visit the fertility clinic, you will be given a physical examination, swabs may be taken from the cervix to rule out the presence of infection, and you will be advised to undergo a test to make sure your fallopian tubes are open.

Checking the Fallopian Tubes

There are two ways of checking the fallopian tubes. The simplest way is to perform an X ray called a *hysterosalpingogram* (HSG), which is performed by a radiologist within 10 days of either a natural or artificially induced period (to rule out the risk of a pregnancy). X-ray dye is gently injected through the cervix, and X-ray pictures are taken to provide an outline of the inside of the uterus and also of the fallopian tubes.

If any abnormalities appear on the HSG, or if you have a history of gynecological problems, you may be advised to undergo a laparoscopy. A laparoscopy is an operative procedure performed under general anesthetic in which a scope is passed through a small incision just below the navel. Through the scope the surgeon can see all the pelvic structures and assess the uterus, fallopian tubes, and ovaries. It should be possible to deal with simple problems at the time of the initial laparoscopy, such as adhesions (scar tissue) around the ovaries and tubes caused by previous infection or endometriosis. Sometimes it is necessary to perform more extensive surgery at a later date.

Stimulating Ovulation

For induction of ovulation to be successful, it is important that the fallopian tubes and pelvic organs be healthy and that sperm function be normal. If significant problems are detected during these baseline investigations, it may be necessary to proceed straight to in vitro fertilization (IVF; see below).

Before induction of ovulation, you may be advised to undergo a glucose tolerance test (see Chapter 3). If you are overweight, you may be referred to a dietician, and you may also be advised to take metformin (see Chapter 3). The most commonly used drug to stimulate ovulation is clomiphene citrate (brand name Clomid), an antiestrogen hormonal preparation that stimulates the release of FSH by the pituitary gland. Clomiphene citrate should be taken in the early days of the menstrual cycle (usually during days two through six). If you are not having regular periods, you may be given a short course of a progestogen, such as medroxyproges-terone acetate (brand name Provera), in order to induce an artificial bleed—after first taking a pregnancy test to ensure that you are not pregnant.

Clomiphene citrate achieves ovulation in about 80 percent of women, but as with all fertility therapies, pregnancy does not necessarily occur right away. It is important to understand that, even for optimally fertile couples in their mid-20s, the best chance of a spontaneous pregnancy in one month is about 25 percent; after six months, the chance rises to about 60 percent. After one year, approximately 85 percent of couples will have conceived. Fertility therapies rarely prove better than this natural, cumulative chance of conception over time; moreover, such therapies are usually given to couples who are in an older age group and who therefore have an age-related reduced chance of pregnancy.

With clomiphene citrate the chance of conception is about 40–50 percent after six months, and it rises slowly thereafter. The risk of multiple pregnancy is about 10 percent. The starting dose for clomiphene citrate is 50 mg a day; this may be increased to 100 mg if the lower dose fails to provide satisfactory results. Once regular ovulation is achieved, the therapy may be continued for six months. Then it should be reviewed and sometimes continued, but not for longer than nine to 12 months.

Clomiphene citrate therapy must be monitored by regular ultrasound scan in order to:

◆ ensure that a response is occurring

◆ ensure that the timing of intercourse coincides with ovulation

◆ help to reduce the risk of multiple pregnancy

Clomiphene citrate therapy will generally be administered by a fertility clinic that has appropriate facilities that can provide ultrasound monitoring.

An alternative to clomiphene citrate is tamoxifen, which works in the same way (as an antiestrogen preparation). The side effects of both of these drugs include hot flushes, abdominal discomfort, and blurred vision. In the short term, reversible hair loss is occasionally experienced.

If ovulation does not occur in response to clomiphene citrate treatment, the next options are either gonadotrophin therapy or laparoscopic ovarian diathermy. If, on the other hand, ovulation occurs but a pregnancy does not result, the next step is usually to move on to assisted conception in the form of IVF.

Gonadotrophin therapy involves the daily injection of hormone preparations containing FSH. FSH can be purified from the urine of postmenopausal women, where it is found in high concentrations along with LH. These two hormones are the two ingredients in human menopausal gonadotrophin (hMG), which is available these days in a number of different formulations. An alternative is genetically engineered (or "recombinant") FSH. The injections are usually given just under the skin (subcutaneously); you can be taught how to administer them yourself. Some preparations require deeper, intramuscular injections. The starting dose is usually 50–75 units a day; it may be increased or decreased depending on the response.

Gonadotrophin therapy requires very careful monitoring because the numerous follicles within the polycystic ovary are sensitive to stimulation. Once the threshold dose has been reached, the ovaries may almost explode into action, producing far more growing follicles than the single one needed to produce the required egg. Ultrasound monitoring is usually commenced after one week of injections, and then scans are performed every two to three days until the largest follicle has reached a size of 17–18 millimeters (about 0.7 inches). An injection of human chorionic gonadotrophin (hCG) is then given to trigger the release of the egg. Because of the risk of multiple pregnancy, the hCG injection should be withheld if there are three or more follicles larger than 14 mm (0.55 inches).

In one study, the number of pregnancies achieved after ovarian stimulation with gonadotrophins reached 62 percent after six months and 73 percent after 12 months.[14] In the same study, live births reached 54 percent after six months and 62 percent after 12 months.

Women with PCOS are at risk of developing a rare but serious condition called *ovarian hyperstimulation syndrome*, in which too many follicles are stimulated. Because the condition may result in abdominal distension, discomfort, nausea, vomiting, and sometimes difficulty breathing, close monitoring is essential. Sometimes hospital admission may even be required.

As stated above, an alternative to gonadotrophin is laparoscopic ovarian diathermy (LOD), also known as "ovarian drilling." This procedure is performed under general anesthesia; it is similar to the laparoscopic assessment of the pelvis (see above). The aim is to cause four small burns on each ovary; somewhat surprisingly, this appears to kick start the ovary into action. If ovulation fails to occur right away, the ovaries often become more receptive to clomiphene citrate or gonadotrophin therapy. LOD has taken the place of the procedure known as "wedge resection," a more serious operation in which a large part of the ovary is removed in order to make the overall size of it more normal. The problem with wedge resection involved the loss of eggs and the potential for significant scarring around the ovaries and fallopian tubes. LOD, however, also carries all the inherent risks of a surgical operation conducted under general anesthesia.

After six cycles of gonadotrophin therapy, the success rates are better than they are at six months after LOD. By twelve months, however, the results of the two treatments are similar. The greatest success rates for LOD are in women who have lived with a shorter duration of infertility (less than three years) and in those with an elevated level of LH. The advantages of LOD include the reduced risk of multiple pregnancy and the reduced need for monitoring. In practical terms, LOD is usually best for women who find it difficult to attend a clinic for regular and frequent scans, and for those who persistently overrespond to gonadotrophin therapy.[15]

IVF

When ovarian stimulation is unsuccessful, many women resort to in vitro fertilization. Success rates of IVF depend very much on individual characteristics such as age, length of infertility, and body weight. Because ovarian stimulation and IVF are less successful if a woman is seriously overweight, most fertility specialists encourage weight loss before the commencement of therapy. Metformin (see Chapter 3) may be of benefit when combined with fertility treatments. Much research is currently under way to assess the true role of IVF in PCOS.

The process of IVF involves a more complex regimen of drug therapy than is the case in the straightforward induction of ovulation. Each clinic varies slightly in its protocols; you will be given detailed information and an opportunity to talk things through with a doctor and possibly with a counselor. Drugs may be prescribed before ovarian stimulation is started. These drugs sometimes include the combined oral contraceptive pill to regulate the menstrual cycle, a course of GnRH (nafarelin) to switch off the pituitary gland, and then FSH or hMG to stimulate the ovaries.

On average, ovarian stimulation takes 9 to 10 days. At that point an hCG injection is given at night when the follicles have reached the prerequisite size. Collection of eggs is performed 36 hours later, while the woman is mildly sedated. Under ultrasound vision, a needle is guided through the vagina into the ovaries to draw out the eggs (oocytes) from the follicles. The eggs are placed in an incubator in the laboratory with sperm that were produced the same day. If there is a problem with the sperm, then one sperm may be injected into each egg, a procedure called *intercytoplasmic sperm injection*. After two days in the incubator, two or more embryos are transferred into the uterus through the cervix in a procedure that is rather like undergoing a Pap smear. Progesterone pessaries (vaginal suppositories) are then usually taken daily until the results of a pregnancy test are known, which will happen about two weeks later.

Extensive research has shown that the drugs used during IVF appear to be safe, although some women may experience side effects such as headaches, hot flushes, mood swings, tender breasts, and a sore abdomen. There is also a risk of ovarian hyper-stimulation syndrome (see above).

In cases where the hormones administered fail to produce the desired result, it may be possible to alter the dosages and try again during the next menstrual cycle. The success rate of IVF is about 25–30 percent per cycle, depending on a number of factors. The chances of a healthy birth increase to 60 percent after six completed cycles of treatment. Each time pregnancy fails to occur, women and their partners generally experience feelings of intense disappointment, grief, and anger, as well as a sense of failure. It is a good idea for patients to use all the stress-management techniques available to them during this difficult time. Most fertility clinics have a trained counselor on staff who will offer to discuss patients' feelings with them after each failed attempt. The counselor understands that this is a difficult time for both partners that is likely to put enormous strain on the relationship (see Chapter 7 for information on emotional support).

A number of factors are now recognized as influencing the possibility of achieving a pregnancy during IVF. These include maintaining a stable weight, eating a balanced diet, and control-ling stress. Indulging in a few sessions of a complementary therapy that you find enjoyable, such as aromatherapy massage or reflexol-ogy treatment, can help to keep your stress levels down.

Chapter 5

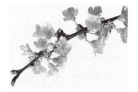

Helping Yourself

There is no doubt that medications can play an important role in controlling the symptoms of PCOS and that they can be invaluable in achieving a pregnancy. However, PCOS is a lifelong condition that invariably responds better when self-help steps are taken by the patient to manage it. The long-term health risks of PCOS are often minimized when the sufferer takes her health into her own hands.

Improving Your Diet

It is now clear that the symptoms of PCOS can be exacerbated by stress, a poor diet, and environmental toxins. Some experts believe that a woman who is genetically predisposed to developing the condition can actually trigger the disorder by indulging in a high-fat diet that contains lots of stimulants (such as caffeine, sugar, and alcohol) and by combining that diet with exposure to certain environmental chemicals. However, evidence indicates that cutting down on saturated fats and stimulants can reduce the symptoms.

After seeing your doctor, making dietary improvements should ideally be the second step in your journey toward better health. Eating more healthily may not be a cure for PCOS, but it can help to reduce the symptoms. It can also help to minimize the long-term health risks associated with the condition.

In general, the quality of people's diets has deteriorated over the past several decades. Crops are now loaded with artificial chemicals, and once the foods are harvested, more chemicals are added to allow them to travel long distances and to withstand a long shelf life (i.e., to keep them looking fresh and to enhance their flavor). However, foods that have been refined and processed in this way hold little nutritional value, and the chemical content is known to be harmful to health.[16] As a consequence, we constantly ingest low levels of toxins, which are likely to upset the hormone levels within the body. Since hormone levels in PCOS are already abnormal, further disturbance may only exacerbate the situation.

The following points summarize the current eating habits of most residents of industrialized nations:

- We eat food that has been sprayed multiple times with chemical pesticides, herbicides, and fungicides. These poisons kill essential soil microbes that would otherwise help plants to absorb nutrient-rich minerals (such as zinc, copper, magnesium, and manganese) that are essential to good health.

- We eat food grown on land that has been artificially fertilized with nitrogen, potassium, and phosphorous instead of with manure or compost. Although artificial fertilizers stimulate plant growth, their use has greatly reduced the mineral content of soil. This also causes an imbalance in our hormone levels. Organically grown foods may be a little more expensive, but they are free of toxins and they taste good.

- Plant foods are typically ripened, stored, and processed using artificial processes. The refining and storage processes rob foods of the majority of their fiber and nutrients. Vitamin E and most of the precious B vitamins are lost in the processing and bleaching of wheat and flour, leaving it free of nutritional value. Similarly, all other grains, fruits, and vegetables lose many of their nutrients during processing, especially vitamin C, which is highly vulnerable to processing of any sort.

◆ We eat only the tasty parts of the food, disposing of the rest. For example, wheat husks and wheat germ—the most nutritious parts of the plant—are removed before the remaining grain is processed into white flour. By contrast, "whole" foods contain fiber, which is important in aiding the removal of waste materials from the intestines. Eating foods naturally high in fiber is vital to good bowel health.

Eliminating Food Additives from Your Diet

Eliminating additives, such as food colorings, preservatives, and flavorings, should ensure that the toxicity that interferes with our hormone levels is reduced. Doing so can even go some way toward helping to rebalance hormone levels in the body.

Unfortunately, the majority of the foods on our supermarket shelves have undergone some degree of chemical refinement or alteration. The additives that cause the most harm are monosodium glutamate (MSG), artificial colorings, butylated hydroxyanisole (BHA), butylated hydroxytoluene (BHT), sorbate, sulfites, and aspartame (NutraSweet).

Contrary to popular belief, aspartame may not help you to lose weight. It is known to trigger a craving for carbohydrate, which can cause a person to put on weight. Aspartame is commonly found in foods described as "low sugar," "sugar free," or "diet."

What Should Women with PCOS Eat?

Eating a well-balanced, organic, whole-food diet can be of great benefit to women with PCOS. At first it may be difficult to make the recommended dietary changes, but the benefits to your overall health will make the effort worthwhile. However, if you find you are unable to make great changes, don't feel guilty or despondent. Small changes are better than no changes at all, and even small changes will make a difference.

Reducing Sugar and Refined Carbohydrates

Our diets today are often high in sugar and refined carbohydrates (which are found in cookies, cakes, pastries, and so on). Refined carbohydrates cause a rapid rise in blood glucose levels. When we consistently consume high levels of sugar and refined carbohydrates, our bodies make an excess of insulin, which, as we have discussed, can be detrimental to women with PCOS, causing an increase in weight and exacerbating the symptoms. Furthermore, these types of foods hold little nutritional value, and digesting, absorbing, and eliminating these types of foods uses up a great deal of the body's energy.

Sugar—which has been dubbed "the scourge of the age"—contains no nutritional value whatsoever (besides calories). In fact, sugar consumption has been linked with many disorders, from diabetes to heart disease and cancer. You probably know that sugar converts into energy. However, you may not know that we can actually obtain all the sugars and energy we need from fruit and complex (unrefined) carbohydrates such as lentils and whole grains. These unrefined carbohydrates are converted into sugar in the body as nature intended.

Reducing Salt

Salt is commonly used as a preservative and a flavor enhancer; it is added to most processed, prepackaged foods. Most breakfast cereals, for example, are high in salt. As a result, people who eat a lot of processed foods may be consuming more salt than they realize, especially when the salt used in cooking and at the table is also taken into account. By contrast, whole foods actually contain salt (sodium) and potassium in just the right balance for our bodies.

Adding extra salt to our foods upsets this happy balance and can lead to a variety of problems. Try using herbs and spices (in moderation) for flavoring. Sea salt contains more minerals than ordinary salt, but it is still salt—so use it sparingly.

Reducing Red Meat and Dairy Products

Saturated fats from dairy products and red meat are recommended only in moderation for women with PCOS. These fats can stimulate the body to produce too much estrogen and prostaglandins, and a woman with PCOS already has an excess of these hormones. In addition, consumption of red meat slows down the waste-elimination process, causing the body to reabsorb estrogen that has become compacted in the bowels.

White meat and fish—particularly oily fish such as herring, mackerel, sardines, salmon, and tuna—are good sources of protein and health-promoting oils. Refrain from eating portions of meat or fish that are larger than the palm of your hand. When you buy the meat of land-dwelling animals, try to ensure that you buy only organic meat—that is, from animals reared without the use of antibiotics, anabolic steroids, chemical pesticides in their feed, etc.

Reducing Caffeine

Caffeinated products, which include coffee, tea, cocoa, cola drinks, and chocolate, cause stress to the adrenal glands. In excess, they are also toxic to the liver and can reduce the body's ability to absorb vitamins and minerals. If caffeine is consumed regularly in fairly high quantities, it is likely to give rise to chronic anxiety, the symptoms of which are agitation, palpitations, headaches, indigestion, panic, insomnia, and hyperventilation. Drinking more than two cups of coffee a day has been linked to the development of endometriosis.[17] The best advice you can receive is to remove caffeinated products from your diet.

Unfortunately, the addictive nature of caffeine makes reduction far from easy. Withdrawal symptoms can take the form of splitting headaches, fatigue, depression, poor concentration, and muscle pains. It is no wonder that people feel terrible until they have had their first dose of caffeine in the morning and can't seem to function properly without regular doses throughout the day! Fortunately, caffeine is quickly "washed out" of the system, and it is possible to minimize withdrawal symptoms by slowly reducing your intake over several weeks.

A problem for many women is finding an acceptable alternative to caffeinated beverages. Coffee, tea, cocoa, and cola drinks can be replaced by fruit and vegetable juices and herbal teas. Green tea is an excellent alternative, as is rooibosch (redbush) tea. Be aware that green tea contains caffeine; however, the stimulating effect of the caffeine appears to be counteracted by the beneficial ingredients contained in green tea. Both green tea and redbush tea are low in tannin and high in antioxidants. A variety of grain-based coffee substitutes may be purchased at natural-foods stores, but they are not a good choice as a substitute for traditional caffeinated products because many decaffeinated products are processed with the use of chemicals.

Carob, which is similar to the cocoa bean, is a healthy, caffeine-free alternative to cocoa and chocolate. It contains less fat and is naturally sweet, unlike the cocoa bean, which is bitter and needs sweetening. Many people find carob bars an enjoyable replacement for chocolate bars and other candy. Carob is also available in powder form for use in baking and in drinks.

Dietary Fats

Fats (fatty acids) are the most concentrated sources of energy in our diet. One gram of fat provides the body with nine calories of energy. Compare this with the other dietary substances that contain calories: carbohydrates and protein, which each provide four calories per gram, and alcohol, which provides seven calories per gram.

As you are probably aware, some types of fat are beneficial to health, whereas other types are capable of raising cholesterol levels and consequently causing health problems. Fats can be categorized into two main types—saturated fat and unsaturated fat.

Saturated fat is believed to be implicated in the development of heart disease. It comes mainly from animal sources and is generally solid at room temperature (e.g., butter). Although margarine was believed to be a healthier choice than butter for many years, nutritionists have now revised their opinion. This is because some of the fats involved in the processing of margarine are changed into hydrogenated oils (also known as trans-fatty acids), which the body metabolizes as if they were saturated fatty acids—the same as the fats contained in butter. Bottom line: Trans-fatty acids are just as bad for people's health as saturated fats. Avoid them by steering clear of food products that list "partially hydrogenated vegetable oils" on their labels. Butter is a valuable source of oils and vitamin A, but should be used sparingly. Margarine, on the other hand, is an artificial product that contains many additives.

Unsaturated fat, also called polyunsaturated or monounsaturated fat, has a protective effect on the heart and other organs. Unsaturated fat is usually liquid at room temperature. Omega-3 and omega-6 oils, both unsaturated fatty acids, occur naturally in oily fish, nuts, and seeds. It is recommended that women with PCOS eat oily fish at least three times a week and consume cold-pressed oils such as olive oil, canola oil, safflower oil, and sunflower oil daily, in salad dressings and in cooking. Of these, olive oil is best suited to cooking, because it suffers less damage from heat than other oils.

Frying

The process of frying changes the molecular structure of foods, rendering them potentially damaging to the body. If you must fry something, it is best to use a small amount of extra-virgin olive oil and to cook it at a low temperature. A healthier alternative is to sauté the food in a little water or tomato juice, or to grill, bake, or steam it. Stir-frying is good—but cook the food in a little water, drizzling on the olive oil afterwards.

Remember that used oils should never be reheated. Doing so can be harmful to the body. Also, oils should be stored in sealed containers in a cool, dark place to prevent rancidity.

Eggs

You are no doubt aware that eggs are high in cholesterol, which when consumed in excess can harm the cardiovascular system. However, eggs also contain lecithin, which is a superb biological "detergent" that is capable of breaking down fats so they can be utilized by the body—an ability that makes lethicin very helpful to women with PCOS. Lecithin also prevents the accumulation of too many acidic or alkaline substances in the blood and encourages the transportation of nutrients through the cell walls. Eggs should be soft-boiled or poached, since a hard yolk binds the lecithin, rendering it useless as a "fat detergent."

Although it is generally recommended that people eat only two or three eggs a week, individuals following a vegetarian diet should eat up to five eggs a week to obtain a sufficient amount of protein.

A Whole-Food Diet

Whole foods are simply those that have had nothing taken away (nutrients or fiber) and that have had nothing added (colorings, flavorings, or preservatives). In short, they are foods in their most natural form. Whole foods that are organically produced, without the use of potentially dangerous chemical fertilizers, pesticides, and herbicides, are even better for us.

The fiber contained in grains, fruits, and vegetables is particularly beneficial for women with PCOS. Fiber reduces estrogen levels by protecting the estrogens secreted in the bile, effectively preventing them from being reabsorbed into the blood. Low-fat, unrefined vegetarian foods are excellent since they help to speed up the transit time of waste products through the large intestine and thus eliminate old estrogens in the bowel.

Below we have outlined many of the foods recommended in a whole-food diet.

Fresh Fruits and Vegetables

As well as helping to eliminate old estrogens in the large intestine, the high levels of fiber in fruits and vegetables also help to regulate insulin levels, as shown in several recent studies. Try to eat locally grown, organic foods that are in season. They have the highest nutrient content and the greatest enzyme activity. Enzymes are to our body what spark plugs are to a car's engine. Without its "sparks," the body doesn't work properly. Organically grown fruit and vegetables may look less perfect than those that have been grown with the use of pesticides and artificial fertilizers, but they *are* superior; foods grown in the conventional method are devitalized of some of their "spark."

Try to eat foods as fresh and as raw as possible. Learn to make a variety of salads, and try to eat one every day. When you do cook vegetables, cook them in a minimum amount of unsalted (or lightly salted) water for the minimum length of time. Lightly steaming or stir-frying are healthy alternatives. Scrub vegetables rather than peel them.

Legumes (Dried Peas and Beans)

Although they contain high amounts of protein, legumes cost very little. The soybean offers complete protein—that is, it contains all the essential amino acids. Soy products can be purchased as soy milk, tofu, tempeh, and miso, to name just a few. Tofu is very versatile and can be used in both savory and sweet dishes.

Because the soybean also contains phytoestrogens—which are plant hormones that help to reduce high estrogen levels (see below)—soy foods are highly recommended for people with PCOS. Butter beans, mung beans, chickpeas, haricot beans, lentils, garden peas, kidney beans, pinto beans, black beans, and split peas are rich sources of phytoestrogens and should be consumed as often as possible.

Seeds

Seeds are not only for the birds! Sunflower, sesame, hemp, and pumpkin seeds contain a wonderful combination of nutrients, all of which are necessary to start a new plant and are also very important for normalizing the body's systems. They can be eaten raw as a snack, sprinkled over salads and cereals, or used in baking. For more flavor they can be lightly roasted and tossed with organic soy sauce. Cracked linseed is highly nutritious and is also useful for treating constipation. It can be used in baking and sprinkled over hot and cold breakfast cereals. Since they contain phytoestrogens, flax, pumpkin, and sesame seeds are particularly beneficial.

Nuts

Nuts, too, should be an intrinsic part of your diet. All nuts contain vital nutrients, but almonds, cashews, Brazil nuts, and pecans offer perhaps the greatest array. Eat a wide assortment of nuts as snacks, with cereals, and in baking. Walnuts are excellent since they are high in phytoestrogens.

Grains

Wheat is our staple grain in the West. Refined wheat flour is the product with which most of our cakes, pastries, cookies, and breads are made. However, refined wheat flour is not actually good for us; "refined" means that the husks and the germ of the wheat have been removed and the remaining powder bleached. As a result, most of the nutritional value is removed, including the vitamins, minerals, protein, and fiber. Only carbohydrates, calories, and a little protein remain.

Fortified flours, as the name implies, have had some of their nutrients replaced. However, vitamin B-6, vitamin E, and folic acid are not put back in during the fortification process. Also, of the nine minerals initially removed during refining, only three—iron, calcium, and phosphorous—are returned, but in forms that are not easily absorbed by the body. All in all, refined flours have little nutritional value.

Healthy flours include whole-wheat flour, spelt flour, quinoa flour, oat flour, maize flour, brown-rice flour, rye flour, barley flour, and potato flour, all of which are high in nutrients. Buckwheat, although not actually a grain, can also be made into a flour that serves as a delicious alternative to refined flour. As with millet and rice, buckwheat is free of gluten, a common allergen. Because wheat germ is high in the B vitamins that are so important to women with PCOS, it is highly recommended. Whole-grain breads, to which crushed wheat, rye grains, and other whole grains have been added, are also a pleasant alternative to goods made from refined flour. Bread mixes that are nutritious and easy to prepare can be purchased in natural-foods markets. Remember that organically produced flours are more nutritious than those that are refined or fortified.

A word of warning: Please ensure that your "whole-grain" loaf of bread really *is* whole-grain and not simply made of dyed white flour or a mixture of white and whole-wheat flours. The word "brown" in the description of a bread tells you nothing.

You should aim to consume a variety of grains. Oats are highly recommended for women with PCOS, as they help to stabilize blood sugar levels.

Phytoestrogens

Phytoestrogens are naturally occurring nutrients in plants that exert an estrogen-like effect on the body (*phyto-* means "plant"). Studies have shown that the chemical structure of phytoestrogens is very close to that of human estrogen. Studies also indicate that although phytoestrogens are less powerful than human estrogens, they can play an important role in the healthy functioning of the human body. For example, if the body's estrogen levels are low, as is the case during menopause, phytoestrogens add to the body's estrogen stores. Alternatively, when estrogen levels are high, as is often the case in PCOS, plant hormones can actually lower the body's estrogen levels. They do this by competing with estrogen for the "binding sites" in the body where estrogen usually exerts its effects.

Scientists have discovered hundreds of edible phytoestrogens. They occur in many different plants, including soybeans, whole grains, fennel, parsley, celery, and flaxseed oil, as well as in many nuts, seeds, and herbs. The herbs known to be particularly useful for women with PCOS because of their phytoestrogen content are black cohosh, red clover, dong quai, licorice, Korean ginseng, and wild American ginseng.

Studies have shown that a phytoestrogen-rich diet can protect against endometrial cancer and can lower cholesterol levels. However, it is important to seek professional advice before taking any herbs during pregnancy.

A Sample Meal Plan

To give you an idea of the types of foods recommended for women with PCOS, we have devised a seven-day sample meal plan (pp. 59–60). If our suggestions are very different from your current diet, please don't be daunted. This is an ideal, something that you might want to aim for over a period of time, and some of the foods can be replaced with equivalents that are more to your taste or more easily available in your area. For those of you desiring additional sample menus, a good source is *The PCOS Diet Book* (see Further Reading).

Beverages are not included in the sample meal plan, but you should consume plenty of water, herbal teas, and fresh fruit and vegetable juices. All fruits and vegetables should be organic, all breads whole-grain, and any prepackaged foods that contain additives should be avoided.

Note that when we say "cup," we mean a standard measuring cup (i.e., eight fluid ounces) rather than a mug.

A Sample Meal Plan for Women with PCOS

Day 1

Breakfast: Grapefruit with a little muscovado sugar and two slices of whole-grain toast (muscovado sugar, a dark brown sugar from India, can be obtained in gourmet or specialty-food stores. It is not the same as American brown sugar but rather richer and more satisfying)

Snack: 1/3 cup mixed sunflower seeds and almonds

Lunch: A salad of your choice, with low-fat mayonnaise or salad dressing but no cheese; an apple

Snack: 1/3 cup dried apricots

Dinner: Stew with lean beef and plenty of vegetables

Snack: Two oatcakes (available from natural-foods stores)

Day 2

Breakfast: Oatmeal or other hot cereal with cracked linseed, raw honey, and rice milk

Snack: Banana

Lunch: Two soft-poached eggs on two slices of whole-grain toast

Snack: 1/3 cup pecans

Dinner: Grilled chicken breast with potatoes, carrots, and green beans

Snack: An apple

Day 3

Breakfast: Grilled sardines on two slices of whole-grain toast

Snack: Carob bar (available from natural-foods stores)

Lunch: Bean and vegetable soup with two whole-grain rolls; a pear

Snack: 1/3 cup mixed dried fruits and nuts

Dinner: Homemade chicken curry with brown rice

Snack: Two slices of whole-grain toast

Day 4

Breakfast: Large wedge of cantaloupe

Snack: Two oat cakes

Lunch: Tuna salad; a banana

Snack: 1/3 cup dried apricots

Dinner: Falafel (similar to a veggie burger and available from natural-foods stores) with beans and homemade oven fries; an orange

Snack: Two cookies

Day 5

Breakfast: Oatmeal or other hot cereal with cracked linseed, rice milk, and a little muscovado sugar

Snack: 1/3 cup pecans

Lunch: Grilled fish fillet with two slices of whole-grain bread

Snack: Two kiwi fruit

Dinner: Mixed vegetable casserole

Snack: Two slices of whole-grain toast with raw honey

Day 6

Breakfast: Fresh fruit salad

Snack: Whole-grain crackers with cottage cheese

Lunch: Chicken broth; an apple

Snack: 1/3 cup mixed nuts

Dinner: Tuna salad with two whole-grain rolls

Snack: An orange

Day 7

Breakfast: Two slices of whole-grain toast with raw honey

Snack: Two rice cakes

Lunch: Mixed salad; baked apples

Snack: A pear

Dinner: Baked wild salmon with potatoes, broccoli, and carrots

Snack: Two oat cakes

Making Changes

Changing the habits of a lifetime takes a lot of effort and determination. Eating is a pleasurable activity; we are used to choosing the foods that satisfy our taste buds (often made more tasty by the addition of chemical flavorings, fat, sugar, salt, and so on), and we may be loath to make drastic changes. For these reasons, it is recommended that you alter your eating habits *gradually*, allowing yourself time to adjust to the new textures, appearances, and flavors of different foods. With perseverance, your tastes *will* change—and as your PCOS symptoms decline, your interest in your new diet will probably increase!

If you wish to start following our recommended food plan right away, we must add a word of warning. Nutritious, cleanly grown foods may trigger the body into instant detoxification, causing headaches, lethargy, and even diarrhea. These symptoms may last from one day to two weeks. You can avoid this shock to your system by changing gradually to healthier foods.

As you introduce the new diet, remember that it is important to eat a wide variety of foods. Eating the same things over and over causes the body to miss out on many vital building blocks; this is because certain nutrients build and regenerate only certain parts of the body.

In comparison with the average Western diet, which, by the addition of chemical flavorings, saturated fat, sugar, and salt, has evolved largely to please the taste buds, a healthy diet is based on foods in their more natural form. It is therefore advisable that you *slowly* retrain your palate to accept different tastes. For this reason, we recommend that you cut back gradually on the amounts of sugar, salt, and saturated fat that you consume. It takes only a month of eating a food regularly for it to become a habit.

If there are foods in the sample diet you just know you won't eat on a regular basis, simply eliminate them from your mind. A long-term diet will only work if it is practical, sustainable, and compatible with your lifestyle. If you feel it is too difficult to practice healthy eating on your own, you may want to ask your doctor for a referral to a dietician or nutritionist for additional help.

Using a Diary to Set Goals

Keeping a food-intake diary is an excellent way to monitor your progress. We suggest that you buy a notebook and devote a page to each day, listing all the foods you eat, including snacks and beverages.

It is a good idea to set small, achievable goals on the very first page of your diary—that way you should be able to get results more quickly. For example, you may wish to set a goal of eating two types of organic vegetables each day. Without the diary, you might assume you have done badly—but when you read your entries you may see that you have actually eaten two types of vegetables two or three times a week. That's a good starting point. Now you can focus on slowly increasing that amount.

Try to avoid making too many changes in too short a time. This is not a fad diet you are trying; it is, we hope, a permanent lifestyle change, a step toward both weight loss (if necessary) and better health. Perhaps after setting a goal of eating more vegetables, you could set another to eat more fruit (again, try to buy only organic fruit). Next, you could try to cut down on soft drinks and coffee and replace them with fruit juice, water, and herbal teas. Cutting down on foods containing additives could be your next goal—with the eventual aim of eliminating these foods from your diet entirely.

One more hint: Try to avoid counting calories. You should soon feel the benefit of your new eating habits in how your clothes fit. You might want to begin saving up for a whole new wardrobe for when you drop a dress size or two! Even if you are not overweight, an improved diet should have a positive impact on your PCOS.

Dietary Supplements for Women with PCOS

Some experts believe that anyone with a health problem is naturally deficient in certain vitamins and minerals. For that reason, women with PCOS may wish to take supplements. Supplements generally come in tablet or capsule form. They can be purchased at natural-foods stores and through specialty suppliers. They should be taken before meals to ensure maximum absorption. Look for supplements without added colorings, flavorings, preservatives, hydrogenated fats, gelatin, and sugar, and compare the dosages contained in different brands of the same supplement. Some supplements contain only minute amounts of the active ingredients. A good company will have a qualified nutritionist available to answer telephone queries and will train retailers to be knowledgeable about their products. Of course, some retailers may still be biased toward their own products.

Supplements for women with PCOS include the following:

◆ *Chromium.* Studies have shown that chromium supplementation can improve glucose tolerance and the efficiency of insulin. Women with PCOS may wish to take up to 0.2 mg daily.

◆ *B vitamins.* These are known to help relieve stress. This helps to detoxify the hormones that are to be secreted from the body. Women with PCOS may wish to take up to 25 mg daily.

◆ *A good antioxidant multivitamin-mineral combination.* Antioxidants clean up the harmful "free radicals" in our bodies that come from sources such as industrial pollutants, ultraviolet light leaking through the ozone layer, car exhaust fumes, and smoking. They help the body at the important cellular level. Follow the dosage instructions on the label.

◆ *Zinc.* This mineral, another antioxidant, aids in the maintenance of the reproductive organs. It also helps to correct insulin levels. Women with PCOS may wish to take up to 30 mg daily.

◆ *Evening primrose oil*. This essential fatty acid contains gamma-linolenic acid, which aids hormone balance. Women with PCOS may wish to take 500–1,000 mg daily.

Water

Because water is required for most of the reactions in our bodies, a steady intake is essential (at least eight glasses a day). However, whether tap water is fit for human consumption is a matter for debate. Aluminum sulfate is added as a coagulant to groundwater, then chemical polyelectrolytes are added to further settle the coagulated waste. Next, the water is passed through sand filters to remove the settled particles. However, many of the added chemicals remain. The treated groundwater is then combined with reservoir water, to which fluoride and chlorine are added. By the time it reaches our taps, it is loaded with inappropriate mineral salts and added chemicals. Other pollutants also often seep in and contaminate the water further.

Tap water may be of some detriment to people with PCOS, so you may wish to use purified (filtered) water. It has the effect of detoxifying the harmful toxins in the environment and those ingested via processed foods. Water filters on the market vary from simple carbon filters to carbon filters with silver mesh components that even destroy bacteria.

There are also reverse osmosis filters, which produce very clean water while still retaining some of the precious trace minerals. It must be said, however, that a filter's individual effectiveness at removing pollutants is in proportion to its cost. Don't let this put you off, though—an inexpensive carbon filter is far better than no filter at all.

Estrogens in the Environment

Some of the chemicals in our environment are capable of altering hormone levels; they are known collectively as *endocrine-disrupting chemicals*. The result of exposure to these substances can be seen in some of the fish in our rivers whose development has been greatly affected. It has been known for some years that a wide variety of chemicals are capable of disrupting the reproductive system by mimicking natural estrogen, and in fish the effect can be seen when males develop female sexual organs.

It must be assumed that these estrogen mimics have an effect on humans, too. This is seemingly evident in the dramatic drop in the average male's sperm count over the past 50 years. Halfway through the last century the average sperm count was considered to be more than 60 million sperm per milliliter. Today the normal count is defined as above 20 million sperm per milliliter. Furthermore, the incidence of menstrual disturbance, endometriosis, fibroids, infertility, and breast cancer has almost tripled in the past 50 years. It can be assumed that endocrine-disrupting chemicals in the environment are at least partly to blame.

Since processed foods contain endocrine-disrupting chemicals—for example, monosodium glutamate (MSG), butylated hydroxyanisole (BHA), and butylated hydroxytoluene (BHT)—it would be advisable to eat organic foods and to cut down on your exposure to chemicals at home and in the workplace. Many personal-care products also contain endocrine-disrupting chemicals, such as ammonium laurel (or laureth) sulfate, ammonium chloride, and sodium laurel (or laureth) sulfate; however, natural products can now be obtained from natural-foods stores and specialty manufacturers.

Exercise

Since up to 50 percent of the PCOS population is thought to be clinically obese, exercise is just as important as diet in managing the condition. Building up muscle mass and decreasing body fat can have a positive effect on many bodily functions. For instance, a lower body weight and reduced body fat levels will raise levels of SHBG, which is generally low in women with PCOS. A higher level of SHBG is advantageous as it reduces testosterone action.

This, in turn, can decrease the symptoms of hirsutism, acne, and hair loss. Aerobic and weight-bearing exercise have the effect of reducing insulin resistance: Fat and muscle cells react more kindly to insulin in the blood, as a result of which the body needs to pump out less insulin to achieve the same response.

Warming Up

It is important to warm up and mobilize the muscles and joints before embarking on aerobic and weight-bearing exercise. Warming up will prepare the cardiovascular system for a workout by gradually increasing the body temperature and the blood flow to the working areas. A good warm-up also helps to prevent muscular soreness and injury.

Stand with your feet about 15 inches apart, and keep your body relaxed, your back straight, your bottom tucked in, and your stomach muscles contracted as you perform the following routine. Make your movements smooth and continuous.

Shoulders

Letting your arms hang loose, slowly circle your shoulders in a backward motion. Repeat 10 times. Now slowly circle your shoulders forward and repeat this motion 10 times.

Neck

Slowly turn your head to the left and hold for a count of two, then return your head to the center; repeat the exercise 10 times. Next, turn your head to the right and hold for a count of two; return to the center. Repeat 10 times. Tucking in your chin, tilt your head down and hold for a count of two before returning to the center. Repeat 10 times. Finally, tilt your head upward and hold for a count of two before returning to the center. Repeat 10 times.

Spine (first set of warm-ups)

Placing your hands on your hips to help support your lower back and slowly tilt your upper body to the left and hold for a count of two. Be sure to keep your hips centered rather than letting them shift in the direction opposite your upper torso. Return to the center, and repeat between two and 10 times. Now tilt to the right and return to the center. Repeat between two and 10 times (see Figure 3).

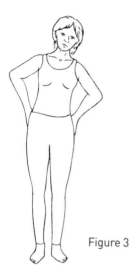

Figure 3

Spine (second set of warm-ups)

Keeping your lower back still, swing your arms and turn your upper body to the left as far as it will comfortably go, then return to the center. Repeat 10 times. Now swing your arms and turn your upper body to the right and return to the center. Repeat 10 times.

Hips and knees

With your torso upright, move your hips by lifting your left knee upward, as far as is comfortable. Hold for a count of two, then lower. Now raise your right knee and hold for a count of two. Repeat 10 times (see Figure 4).

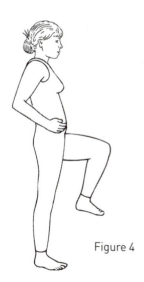

Figure 4

Figure 5

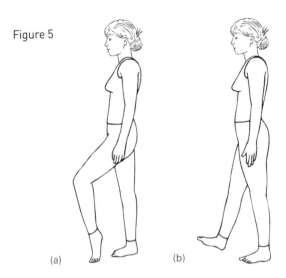

(a)   (b)

Ankles

With your supporting leg slightly bent, place your left heel on the floor in front of you. Now lift your foot, and then place your left toes on the floor. Repeat 10 times. Repeat the exercise with the right foot (see Figure 5).

Pulse-Raising Activities

Pulse-raising activities, another part of your warm-up routine, should gradually increase in intensity. Their purpose is to warm your muscles further in preparation for stretching. March in place for two to four minutes, starting slowly and then gradually increasing your rate.

Stretching Exercises

Stretches prepare the muscles for the more challenging movements that will follow.

Calf (first set of stretching exercises)

Stand with your arms outstretched in front of you at shoulder

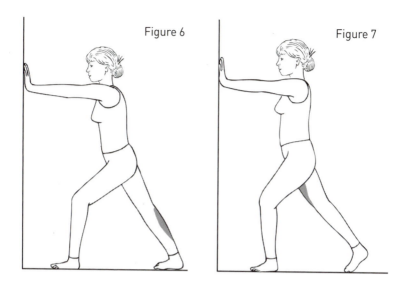

Figure 6   Figure 7

level, palms against the wall. Keeping your left foot on the floor, bend your left knee. Press the heel of your right foot into the floor until you feel a gentle stretch in your leg muscles. Now change legs, alternating between the left and right leg. Repeat 10 times (see Figure 6).

Calf (second set of stretching exercises)

Standing with your feet slightly apart, raise both heels off the floor so that you are on your toes. Repeat 10 times. As your calf muscles strengthen you should be able to stay on your toes for longer periods of time.

Front of thigh (quadriceps)

Using a chair or the wall for support, stand with your left foot about eight inches in front of your right, both knees bent, your right heel off the floor. Tuck in your bottom, and move your hip forward until you feel a gentle stretch in the front of your right thigh. Now change legs. Repeat 10 times (see Figure 7).

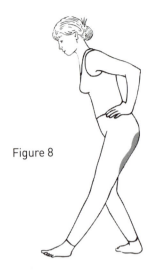

Figure 8

Back of thigh (hamstring)

Stand with your legs slightly bent and your left foot about eight inches in front of your right foot. Keeping your back straight, place both hands on your hips and lean forward a little. Now straighten your left leg, tilting your bottom upward until you feel a gentle stretch in the back of your left thigh. Next, change legs and repeat 10 times (see Figure 8).

Groin

Spreading your legs slightly, with your hips facing forward and your back straight, bend your left leg and slide your right foot slowly sideways, keeping it straight, until you feel a gentle stretch in your groin. Gently move to the right, bending your right leg as you straighten the left (see Figure 9).

Figure 9

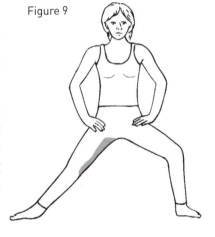

Chest

Keeping your back straight, your knees slightly bent, and your pelvis tucked under, place your hands on the back side of your pelvis as far behind your lower back as you can. Now move your shoulders and elbows back until you feel a gentle stretch in your chest (see Figure 10).

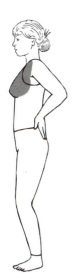

Figure 10

Aerobic Exercise

Aerobic exercise—any activity that increases your heart rate and makes you feel slightly out of breath—should come next. Aerobic exercise is beneficial to women with PCOS since it improves cardiovascular function and helps to protect against high blood pressure (hypertension), heart disease, and stroke. Regular aerobic activity carries the added bonus of releasing "feel-good" endorphins into your bloodstream, hence lifting your mood. It also contributes to overall fitness and aids in the reduction of weight. Try to choose an activity that you will enjoy and want to continue.

Note that you should check with your doctor before embarking on any program of strenuous or regular aerobic activity.

Walking

This most convenient, low-impact aerobic activity aids mobility, strength, and stamina, and helps to protect against osteoporosis. You may find it easier to use a treadmill, which allows you to read a book or magazine while you exercise, or listen to a CD player, the radio, or a book on tape. Try to walk for 20 or 30 minutes. A treadmill should never wholly replace outdoor walking, as sunlight promotes the synthesis of vitamin D. Furthermore, walking outdoors in pleasant surroundings offers a sense of well-being that can't be obtained from walking indoors.

Stepping

Start with a fairly small step (for example, a wide, hefty book, such as a catalogue or a telephone directory); or, if you wish, use a stair-climbing machine or the bottom step of your staircase. First place your left foot, then your right foot on to the book or step. Now step backwards, first with your left foot, then with your right foot. Repeat for two to 10 minutes, then change feet, first placing your right foot on the step, then your left.

Trampoline jogging

Jogging on a small, circular trampoline can provide a good aerobic workout. If you can manage to get into a rhythm, the trampoline will do much of the work for you. Try to jog for 20 to 30 minutes. Small, inexpensive trampolines are available from most exercise-equipment retailers.

Water aerobics

Many people find water aerobics both easy and enjoyable. Because the water supports your body as you exercise, it removes the shock factor, conditioning your muscles with the very minimum of discomfort. The pressure of the water also causes the chest to expand, encouraging deeper breathing and increased intake of oxygen. Rather than exercising alone in a swimming pool, most people prefer to join a water-aerobics class. Most public swimming pools offer water-aerobics classes, some of which are graded according to their degree of difficulty. As with all exercises, water aerobics are only truly beneficial when performed on a regular basis. If you live a long way from a swimming pool, you will probably find yourself attending less and less often; then you may feel angry with yourself for giving up. To minimize feelings of failure, be wary of undertaking activities that may be difficult to participate in on a regular basis.

Swimming

If you enjoy swimming, try to go to the pool once or twice a week and gradually build up the number of laps you swim. Swimming exercises every muscle in the body in a way that causes them very little stress. However, as with water aerobics or joining a gym, it helps to feel confident, before you start, that you will continue the exercise in the long term.

Cycling

Whether you use a stationary bike or an ordinary bicycle, cycling provides an efficient cardiovascular workout. Start by pedaling slowly, and then gradually increase your pedaling speed. At first, limit your sessions to two or three minutes; then build up to 20 or 30 minutes, if possible.

Strength and Endurance Exercises

Strength and endurance exercises develop the muscles and help to raise levels of SHBG. As a result, the production of testosterone should gradually decline. (If at this point in your workout you feel that you have already done enough, run through the warm-up again as a way of cooling down and congratulate yourself for doing something positive to help yourself. Perhaps when you feel more fit you will be able to incorporate strength training into your routine.)

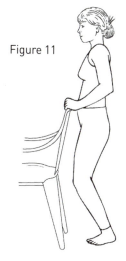

Figure 11

Thighs (first set of strength and endurance exercises)

Lean back against the wall with your feet 12 inches away from the base of the wall. With your posture aligned, slowly squat down, keeping your heels on the ground. Now slowly straighten your legs again. Repeat between two and 10 times.

Thighs (second set of strength and endurance exercises)

Holding on to a sturdy chair and keeping your back "tall," bend and then slowly straighten both legs, keeping your heels on the floor. Repeat the exercise between two and 10 times (Figure 11).

Upper back

Lie face down on the floor. Keeping your legs straight, gently raise your head and shoulders. Hold for a count of two and then lower your head and shoulders. Repeat between two and 10 times (see Figure 12).

Figure 12

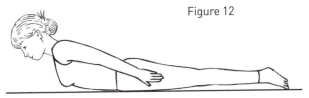

Lower back

Lie on your back and lift your left leg, pulling it toward your chest until you feel a gentle pull in your buttocks and lower back. Repeat with the right leg. Now pull both legs toward your chest at the same time. Repeat each exercise between two and 10 times (see Figure 13).

Figure 13

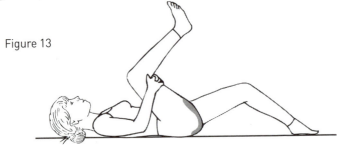

Abdomen

Lie on your back with your knees bent and your feet flat on the floor. Now raise your head and shoulders, reaching with your arms towards your knees. Remember to keep the middle of your back on the floor (see Figure 14).

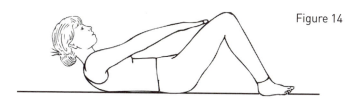

Figure 14

Arms, shoulders, and chest (push-ups)

Stand with your hands flat against a wall, arms straight, body straight, toes about two feet from the wall. Carefully lower your body toward the wall, then slowly push away. Repeat two to 10 times (see Figure 15).

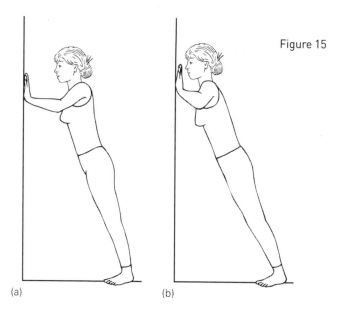

Figure 15

(a)   (b)

Using Weights

Exercising with weights can form a part of your strength and endurance routine and will help you to lose any excess weight. Use either a bag of sugar, a can of food from your pantry, or wrap-around weights that fasten with Velcro around the wrists and ankles. It shouldn't be necessary to use anything heavier.

Fasten the weights around your wrists, or hold a weight firmly in each hand, then stand with your feet slightly apart. Try the following exercises:

- Making sure that only your upper body moves, turn to the left, swinging both arms as you move. To avoid risk of injury, keep the movement controlled (especially the motion of your arms), and don't swing too far. Repeat two to 10 times. Now perform the same exercise and number of repetitions, swinging your body and arms to the right. Ensure that the movements are slow and fluid. Increase the number of repetitions in accordance with your level of fitness.

- Keeping your left elbow close to your waist, slowly raise your left forearm so it almost touches your shoulder. Lower the arm until it is at a right angle to your upper arm, then slowly raise it again. Ensure that your movements are slow and continuous. Repeat between two and 10 times.

- Bend your left arm so that your elbow is near your waist and your forearm is upright (in other words, so that your wrist is at your shoulder), then raise your arm upward until your elbow is straight. Bring it back down to the original position. Repeat once more and then do the same with your right arm. Repeat between two and 10 times.

Cooling Down

Finish your routine by cooling down, using the warm-up exercises described above.

Frequency of Exercise

Ideally, you should follow this routine (or one similar) three or four times a week. Try to exercise before eating breakfast, if possible. The low levels of insulin in your body at that time allow access to body fat for conversion to energy. Remember, too, that every little bit of physical activity helps. To boost your fitness levels further—especially if you are unable to perform a regular aerobic regime—try walking to work, walking to the store, getting off the bus a stop or two earlier, or taking the stairs instead of the elevator.

Managing Stubborn Symptoms

It can be frustrating to feel that you are doing your best to help yourself—taking the prescribed medications and following a healthy diet and exercise program—if you still have to deal with the stubborn, visible effects of PCOS. Unfortunately, it can take up to 18 months for problems like hirsutism, hair loss, and acne to respond to medication, but in the meantime there are things you can do to help manage these symptoms. This section can also benefit those who prefer not to use drug therapy to treat their PCOS.

Unwanted Hair

Several treatments are available for removing unwanted hair. The following information may help you to choose the method most suitable for you.

Electrolysis Treatment

Electrolysis involves a visit to a salon or clinic where a trained electrologist inserts an ultrathin probe into the hair follicle alongside the hair. A small amount of electrical current is delivered to the probe by a device known as an epilator. The electrical current destroys the cells that nourish the hair root, making regrowth weaker with time. Electrolysis is not considered a painful procedure. However, people have different levels of sensitivity, and something that is comfortable for one person can cause discomfort to another. A sensation of some sort is to be expected. Treatment may leave some redness that will last for a few hours.

Some women are referred to a qualified electrologist by their family doctor, endocrinologist, or gynecologist; others rely on the recommendation of a friend or simply look through the local yellow pages. To feel assured you are getting the best treatment, ask your electrologist whether he or she is licensed; licensing is required by law in some states (but not in all). Additionally, two national organizations offer certification programs for electrologists: the American Electrology Association (AEA) and the Society of Clinical and Medical Electrologists (SCME) (see Resources). If your state doesn't require licensing, ask if the electrologist is certified by either of these organizations.

Depilatory Creams

Application of a chemical hair-removal cream (depilatory) causes hair that is visible to dissolve. Be sure to test the cream on a hidden area of skin before using it on the face since depilatories can cause redness and irritation. Some creams may even cause the skin to break out. Depilatories should not be used where acne is present or where the skin is particularly sensitive. If there is persistent acne in the area requiring treatment, electrolysis might be a better option. Depilatory creams remove only the surface hair, making regular application essential. Unfortunately, regrowth is inevitable because the hair root remains intact. The instructions on the label must be carefully followed.

Waxing

Waxing involves hot wax being spread by spatula over the skin. A cloth strip is pressed on to the wax and then pulled off with a quick movement that removes the wax, hair, and dead skin. Yes, it certainly stings! The skin is generally left smooth, but some people suffer redness and bumps, which disappear after a few hours. Because the hair is pulled out by the root, regrowth takes three to eight weeks to become visible. Never apply wax to the nipples when removing hair from the breast area.

Hair should be 1/8 inch long for waxing to be successful. The skin should be pulled taut before the cloth strips are pulled away. Tough hair is easier to remove than fine hair. When waxing facial hair, use the wax at a lower temperature and spread it very thinly. If acne is a problem in the area requiring treatment, wait until the skin has healed before waxing to avoid further irritation. As with depilatory creams, electrolysis is perhaps the best option if acne is persistent. Moreover, if you are taking certain antiacne medications, including tretinoin (brand name Retin-A or Renova), isotretinoin (brand name Accutane), or adapalene (brand name Differin), you are advised to avoid waxing since these medications tend to weaken the skin, causing it to tear when the strips are removed. People with diabetes, poor circulation, or varicose veins should also avoid waxing to remove unwanted hair.

Waxing may be carried out either at a beauty salon or at home with the use of a home waxing kit purchased from a drugstore.

Body sugaring, a procedure offered by some salons, is similar to waxing in that a sugar paste is applied to the skin. However, the paste needs only to be warm, not hot, and it sticks only to the hairs, making removal less painful. Body sugaring also involves less irritation to the skin.

Shaving

Perhaps the easiest option of all, shaving can be used virtually everywhere except the face. Wash the area thoroughly with water as hot as you can bear and use plenty of soap. Shave with a clean blade and try to resist using your partner's razor; shaving with a dull razor is likely to cause reddening and an unsightly rash. Rinse the area thoroughly after shaving. Battery-operated shavers are another option. It is not advisable to shave in sensitive areas, such as around the nipples. Because shavers and razors only remove hair at skin level, regrowth will probably be rapid.

Bleaching

Bleaching is a "concealing" treatment that works well for women whose hair on the head is not too dark. Cream bleaches for facial and body hair are available from drugstores and take only a few minutes to work. Many of these preparations contain aloe vera and vitamin E to soothe the skin. Follow the instructions on the label carefully.

Laser and Photothermolysis

In recent years a great deal of progress has occurred in the use of laser and photothermolysis hair-removal techniques. Both procedures look promising and are much faster and more effective than shaving, waxing, and chemical depilation. Repeated treatments are required for a near-permanent effect because only hair follicles in the growing phase are obliterated at each treatment. Hair growth occurs in three cycles, so six to nine months of regular treatments are typical. Unfortunately, laser and photothermolysis are expensive options and are really suitable only for fair-skinned women with dark hair. This is because depigmentation can occur with darker skin and fair hair is difficult to get at.

Persistent Hair Loss

If your hair is thinning, many cosmetic products are available that can make it appear thicker. If your hair is particularly thin at the crown, choose either a swept-back hairstyle or put your hair up to cover the area. Hair that is receding at the front is more difficult to conceal; in this case, hair-volumizing products may be your best course of action. An improved diet, stress management, drug therapy, or use of the herbal remedy vitex agnus-castus (also known as vitex, chaste tree, chasteberry, or Agnolyt) can promote hair growth. Sometimes it is helpful to wear hair extensions, but they can be costly, and they need to be replaced on a regular basis.

Persistent Acne

If you have a problem with acne that fails to respond to treatment, try the following suggestions:

- ◆ Drink plenty of water. In order to detoxify your system and help the zits retreat, try to drink between six and eight glasses of pure water a day. Distilled water is the best option; however, it is not always readily available. Portable water purifiers, available from supermarkets and many drugstores, can be an inexpensive option. Drinking cool boiled water is another useful alternative.

◆ Eat a well-balanced diet that contains plenty of fruit, vegetables, oily fish, nuts, seeds, and grains.

◆ Tea tree oil can be beneficial, since it contains over 100 natural antifungal, antibacterial, and antiviral properties.

◆ Hemp oil can be useful as a skin cream. It contains omega-6 fatty acids, which have been found to be effective in the treatment of acne.

◆ Sarsaparilla is not only useful for helping to redress a hormonal imbalance, it is also capable of reducing acne.

◆ Echinacea, a natural "antibiotic," can help to improve acne. So can calendula (marigold cream) and goldenseal.

Persistent Difficulty Losing Weight

If you are having difficulties losing weight, consider the following suggestions:

◆ Motivate yourself to follow a balanced diet by telling yourself that not only will you lose weight, but your other PCOS symptoms are likely to improve, too. If you hope to get pregnant, losing weight will increase your chances of conceiving.

◆ Eat plenty of the foods that you are allowed (see the dietary recommendations provided at the beginning this chapter). Remember that saturated fats and refined carbohydrates raise insulin levels and cause fat to be stored in the fat cells. Make sure you keep plenty of healthy snacks on hand. Allow yourself an occasional treat to make the diet easier to cope with.

◆ Get plenty of exercise. Make it a goal to follow an exercise program three or four days a week. Start with a warm-up and go on to strength training and an aerobic activity; you need to slightly increase your heart rate in order for the aerobic portion to be effective (see the exercise program outlined earlier in this chapter). If you really can't face an exercise regime, try as often as you can to walk to and from work, school, or while doing your errands. You will feel pleased with yourself each time you do so. Or, consider joining a fitness class. Some people find exercising in a group more enjoyable than exercising on their own. Most important, increasing your physical activity levels on a regular basis, however you do it, will help you firm your muscles and lose excess fat.

◆ Take a close look at your wardrobe. Keeping "thin" clothes as an incentive to lose weight is unlikely to work. Clothes that are too small are a constant reminder of the weight you've put on; seeing them in your closet is likely to make you feel guilty. Next time you go shopping for clothes take along a friend who is unafraid to speak her mind. Don't necessarily stick to items that feel comfortable; rather, look for clothes that help you to feel feminine, too. Baggy tops can make you appear larger than ever. Try on something that is not exactly clingy, but that skims your figure. You may be pleasantly surprised! Avoid horizontal stripes; choose vertical stripes instead. Women with larger breasts can look top-heavy in high-necked tops. Try something with a lower neckline; you may be surprised at the effect. And why not show off those very feminine assets? Plenty of women would be thrilled to have larger breasts! For ideas, take a look at some of the fashion and beauty magazines that cater specifically to larger women.

◆ Stand proud. Improving your posture, standing tall, and holding back your shoulders can alter other people's impression of you. If you give off an air of confidence, others are more likely to treat you with the respect you deserve. An upright posture also has the effect of making you appear slimmer.

Chapter 6

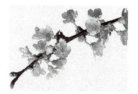

Complementary Treatments

In addition to improving your diet, eliminating endocrine-disrupting chemicals from your environment, and starting an exercise regime, there are many other things women with PCOS can do to help themselves. This chapter discusses treatments that are available in addition to conventional medicine. Collectively, they are called *complementary medicine.*

Organizations that can provide more information about each of the complementary therapies described in this chapter are listed in the Resources. Remember to inform your doctor if you wish to embark on a particular complementary therapy.

What Is Complementary Medicine?

Complementary medicine has been described as "all the therapies not taught in medical school." Complementary therapies include acupuncture, aromatherapy, homeopathy, and reflexology, to name just a few. You may have heard these techniques referred to as "alternative therapies," but that term can be misleading. The word *alternative* suggests they can be used in place of conventional medicine, when that is not the intention. As with treating other disorders, complementary therapies for PCOS should be used in conjunction with the treatment and advice of your own physician. Perhaps one of the main benefits of complementary therapies is that the practitioner is often able to spend time with the patient; thus, she or he can lend more support than a doctor can whose time is stretched thin by a large patient load.

Complementary therapies are suitable for women with PCOS for the following reasons:

- ◆ They are mostly noninvasive.

- ◆ They are mostly free from side effects.

- ◆ They can be used in addition to long-term medication.

- ◆ Most of the therapies are enjoyable; the "patient" can often completely relax, especially in the case of touch and massage techniques.

People who use complementary therapies often report benefits, although this might be partly due to the psychological benefit that comes from knowing they are doing something positive to help themselves. Different therapies seem to suit different people, so consider all of the options that are available to you.

Acupuncture

An ancient form of oriental healing, acupuncture involves puncturing the skin with fine needles at specific points in the body. These points are located along energy channels (called *meridians*) that are believed to correspond to specific internal organs. Needles are inserted to increase, decrease, or unblock the flow of life energy (called *chi*) so the balance between yin and yang is restored.

According to the philosophy behind acupuncture, yin, the female force, is calm and passive; it represents dark, cold, swelling, and moisture. On the other hand, yang, the male force, is stimulating and aggressive, representing heat, light, contraction, and dryness. It is thought that an imbalance in these forces is the cause of illness and disease. A person who always feels cold, suffers from fluid retention, and has fatigue would be considered to have an excess of yin. A person who suffers from headaches and irritation, however, would be deemed to have an excess of yang.

Emotional, physical, or environmental factors are believed to disturb the chi energy balance, and these can also be treated. For example, acupuncture has been used to alleviate stress, digestive disorders, insomnia, asthma, and allergies. In some cases, it is thought to be capable of kick starting menstrual periods and of helping to regulate the menstrual cycle in women with PCOS.

It is thought that there are as many as 2,000 acupuncture points on the body. A qualified acupuncturist will use a set method to determine which acupuncture points need to be treated for any particular condition. During the consultation, the acupuncturist will ask questions about your lifestyle, sleeping patterns, fears, phobias, and reactions to stress. He or she will also ask about your particular health problems and will take your pulse. Then the acupuncture treatments will begin. Women with PCOS can expect to have needles placed at various points in the arms, legs, and abdomen. The acupuncturist will probably work on the liver chi and the spleen chi to treat abnormal bleeding. Some people experience a stinging sensation as the needle goes in; others report feeling little or no discomfort. The first consultation will normally last for an hour; patients should notice improvements after four to six sessions. If no benefits are noted, it may be best to discontinue treatment.

Aromatherapy

Aromatherapy is the utilization of the sense of smell in the treatment of certain health disorders. Aromatherapists work to normalize the hormonal imbalances in PCOS and to aid in relaxation and in the release of emotional stress. Concentrated aromatic oils—also known as essential oils—are extracted from plants and may be inhaled, rubbed directly into the skin, or diluted in water for bathing purposes.

Plant essences have been used for healing throughout the ages; smaller amounts are used for aromatherapy than for herbal medicines. Highly concentrated aromatherapy oils are obtained either by steaming a particular plant extract until the oil glands burst or by soaking the plant extract in hot oil so that the cells collapse and release their essence.

There are three main techniques used in aromatherapy: inhalation, massage, and bathing.

Inhalation of essential oils has a direct influence on the olfactory (nasal) organs, causing the aromas to be received by the brain immediately. In this way, inhalation therapy brings about the quickest results. Steam inhalation is perhaps the most popular technique. Mix a few drops of oil into a bowl of boiling water, or use an oil burner, whereby a tea-light candle heats a small container of water that has a few drops of oil mixed in.

Essential oils intended for massage are normally prediluted. These oils should never be applied directly to the skin in an undiluted (pure) form. When using undiluted essential oils, mix three or four drops with a neutral carrier oil, such as olive oil or safflower oil. The oils penetrate the skin and are absorbed by the body, exerting a positive influence on a particular organ or set of tissues.

Tension and anxiety can also be reduced by using specific aromatherapy oils in the bath. A few drops of pure essential oil should be added directly to running tap water. It disperses and mixes more efficiently this way. No more than 20 drops of oil should be added to bath water.

The oils thought to be particularly useful for women with PCOS are listed below. Each oil can be used in the bath or in a burner, or else mixed with a carrier oil and massaged into the skin.

- *Lavender* is the most popular oil for use in the bath. It is a wonderful restorative and excellent for relieving tension headaches as well as stress.

- *Ylang-ylang* has relaxing properties. It has a calming effect on the heart rate and can be used to relieve palpitations and elevated blood pressure.

- *Chamomile* can be very soothing. It aids both sleep and digestion, and it has anti-inflammatory properties.

- *Jasmine* is a renowned aphrodisiac and can reawaken passion and ease sexual problems. It encourages the expression of pleasure and affection. Because of its powerful aroma, use it in small doses.

◆ *Bergamot* lifts the spirits and can help relieve feelings of depression, anxiety, and insomnia. Its nature is to balance the body and instill composure. If using it as a massage oil, do not apply it before exposure to the sun as doing so may cause irritation to sensitive skin.

◆ *Cedar* gives strength at times of crisis. It calms and soothes nervous tension and anxiety. Its nature is to remind us of our inner strength. Avoid cedar oil during pregnancy.

◆ *Rose* oil is said to bring warmth to the soul. It helps to heal emotional wounds and restores the trust that makes it possible for us to love ourselves.

◆ *Sandalwood* oil acts as a gentle sedative that has an uplifting effect on the psyche.

Because aromatherapy is a holistic treatment (meaning the practitioner considers the person and their ills as a whole), the aromatherapist will ask question about lifestyle, family circumstances, and so on. Depending on your answers, a suitable essential oil (or more than one oil) will be recommended. As well as being beneficial to your health, aromatherapy massages can be very relaxing.

If you prefer the do-it-yourself route, a natural-foods market may be able to provide you with further details about the essential oils that are appropriate to your needs. In addition, you may wish to borrow a good aromatherapy book from the library.

Bach Flower Remedies

In the 1930s, a London doctor named Edward Bach (pronounced "batch") espoused the opinion that "a healthy mind ensures a healthy body." He was a man far ahead of his time, considering it has only been in recent years that we have concluded that the mind and body are closely linked.

Dr. Bach devised a method of treating the negative emotional state behind any disorder. First, he divided emotional states into seven major groups, then he categorized 38 negative states of mind under each group. Using his knowledge of homeopathy, he formulated a plant-based or flower-based remedy to treat each negative state of mind. For example:

1. Fear

For terror he formulated "rock rose" remedy.

For fear of known things he formulated "mimulus."

For fear of mental collapse he formulated "cherry plum."

For fears and worries of unknown origin he formulated "aspen."

For fear or overconcern for others he formulated "red chestnut."

2. Loneliness

For impatience he formulated "impatiens."

For self-centeredness/self-concern he formulated "heather."

For pride and aloofness he formulated "water violet."

3. Insufficient interest in present circumstances

For apathy he formulated "wild rose."

For lack of energy he formulated "olive."

For unwanted thoughts or mental arguments he formulated "white chestnut."

For lack of interest in the present he formulated "clematis."

For deep gloom with no known origin he formulated "mustard."

For failure to learn from past mistakes he formulated "chestnut bud."

For living in the past he formulated "honeysuckle."

4. Despondency or despair

For extreme mental anguish he formulated "sweet chestnut."

For self-hatred or a sense of uncleanliness he formulated "crab apple."

For overresponsibility he formulated "elm."

For lack of confidence he formulated "larch."

For self-reproach or guilt he formulated "pine."

For aftereffects of shock he formulated "star of Bethlehem."

For resentment he formulated "willow."

For those feeling exhausted but struggling on he formulated "oak."

5. Uncertainty

For hopelessness and despair he formulated "gorse."

For despondency he formulated "gentian."

For indecision he formulated "scleranthus."

For uncertainty as to the correct path in life he formulated "wild oat."

For the seeker of advice and confirmation from others he formulated "cerato."

For "Monday morning" blues he formulated "hornbeam."

6. Oversensitivity to influences and ideas

For weak will and subserviency he formulated "centaury."

For mental torment behind a brave face he formulated "agrimony."

For hatred, envy, or jealousy he formulated "holly."

For protection from change and outside influences he formulated "walnut."

7. Overcare for the welfare of others

For intolerance he formulated "beech."

For overenthusiasm he formulated "vervain."

For self-repression/self-denial he formulated "rock water."

For the selfishly possessive he formulated "chicory."

For dominance and inflexibility he formulated "vine."

In addition, Bach's famous "rescue remedy" is appropriate to many everyday situations in which emotional upheaval occurs. It is made from a combination of five Bach flower remedies (rock rose, clematis, cherry plum, impatiens, and star of Bethlehem).

Place a few drops of your chosen remedy on your tongue, or dilute it in water.

Herbal Remedies

Traditional Chinese herbal remedies have been used, to great effect, since antiquity—and they are still the most widely used medicines in the world. In fact, 30 percent of modern conventional medicines are made from plant-derived substances. However, because conventional medicines frequently have toxic side effects, herbal medicines are preferred by many people. Indeed, they seem to rate among the most popular complementary therapies for women with PCOS.

Although they are natural, herbal medicines should be used with caution because they are capable of interacting with prescribed medications. You should always inform your doctor of any herbal preparations you are taking or want to try, *especially if you are on any prescription medications*. Indeed, many doctors believe that herbal medicines should not be taken without the advice of a trained herbalist.

Your chosen herbalist will check your pulse rate and the color of your tongue for clues as to which bodily organs are depleted of energy. He or she will write a prescription for very precise dosages according to your needs. Tablets made from compressed herbal extracts are often supplied, but sometimes patients are given a bag of carefully weighed and ground dried roots, flowers, bark, and other substances, together with full instructions for preparing them and taking them.

Various herbs are considered useful for treating PCOS. They are described below. Please note, however, that no randomized scientific studies large enough to be considered definitive have been undertaken to assess the validity of these claims.

Vitex Agnus-Castus

Vitex agnus-castus (also known as vitex, chaste tree, chasteberry, or Agnolyt) has a long history of use for female hormone regulation. Its apparent effectiveness lies in the fact that it works on the pituitary gland, which stimulates the hormones involved in reproduction. Unlike most other herbal formulations, this remedy is made from the fruit of the plant *Agnus castus* rather than from other parts of the shrub, a fact that seems to contribute to its effectiveness. When it's taken for six to eight months, vitex appears to be capable of stimulating the pituitary gland enough to normalize the menstrual cycle, increasing levels of progesterone and LH and balancing progesterone and estrogen production. This can result in making pregnancy achievable.

Vitex is a member of the family of adaptogenic herbs, which means they are able to adapt to the particular needs of the body. Important note: Taking too much of this herb can cause depression. PCOS patients should start with 30 drops once a day in the morning, and reduce the dosage to 25 or even 20 drops if they start to feel low. Vitex can be obtained either from natural-foods stores or from specialty supplement manufacturers.

Rhodiola Rosea

Rhodiola rosea is a powerful herb native to Russia. It also belongs to the family of adaptogenic herbs. For people who feel stressed, rhodiola can encourage the body to adapt. Research has shown that rhodiola can boost sexual function, help to raise energy levels, increase resistance to disease, and aid in the detoxification of hormones before they are eliminated from the body. It is also believed to have revitalizing properties and to help stabilize mood swings.

Most natural-foods stores now stock this stress-busting adaptogen, as do specialty supplement manufacturers.

Ashwagandha

Ashwagandha (sometimes called *Indian ginseng*), another adaptogenic herb, is an important tonic. It offers a broad range of important healing powers rare in the plant kingdom. Not only is it good for restoring energy in people who often feel tired, but also it has also been shown in research to help ease insomnia and stress.

In one study of 101 subjects, the indications of aging—such as graying hair and low calcium levels—were found to be significantly improved in those taking ashwagandha.[18] Seventy percent of the subjects also reported increased libido and sexual function.

Ashwagandha can be found in most natural-foods stores and is available from specialty supplement manufacturers.

Siberian Ginseng

The many benefits of Siberian ginseng—the most well known of the adaptogenic herbs—are said to include increased physical endurance under stress, improved hormone activity, and better sexual function. This very safe herb is available from most natural-foods stores and specialty supplement manufacturers.

Sarsaparilla

Sarsaparilla is useful for helping to redress a hormonal imbalance. It contains a steroidlike substance that acts in a similar way to progesterone in the body. It is believed to stimulate the reproductive organs and to have a toniclike effect on the sex organs. Sarsaparilla is also capable of reducing acne.

White Peony

White peony is useful for women with PCOS since it can help to normalize androgen levels in the body. It is also thought to reduce irritability and stress.

Echinacea

One of the most widely researched of all the herbs, echinacea has broad antibiotic properties, much like penicillin, and therefore can be useful for treating acne. Alcohol-free tinctures are now available in most natural-foods stores.

St. John's Wort

St. John's wort is probably the most successful natural antidepressant. Studies have shown that it works by increasing the action of the chemical serotonin and by inhibiting depression-promoting enzymes. Similar effects are created by drugs such as fluoxetine (brand name Prozac) and phenelzine (brand name Nardil), which carry a high risk of side effects. St. John's wort, by contrast, has the happy advantage of being virtually free of side effects. (In some cases it can produce an upset stomach, but this reaction should stop within a few days.)

One study has indicated that St. John's wort encourages sleep, and another that it benefits the immune system. In Germany, this herb outsells Prozac by three to one, and is said to be just as effective for treating mild depression. Because of its anti-inflammatory and antiviral properties, it can be useful for treating acne. It helps fight viral infections, too.

Because your skin may be more sensitive to the sun's rays when you are taking St. John's wort, don't forget to use a good sunscreen.

Other Herbal Remedies

German chamomile, lavender, lemon balm, and vervain are other effective herbal remedies that can ease emotional stress.

Homeopathy

The homeopathic approach to medicine is holistic; in other words, the overall health of a person—physical, emotional, and psychological—is assessed before treatment commences. The homeopathic belief is that the whole makeup of a person determines the disorders to which he or she is prone and the symptoms that are likely to occur. After a thorough consultation, the homeopath will offer a remedy compatible with the patient's symptoms as well as with her or his temperament and characteristics. Consequently, two people with the same disorder may be offered entirely different remedies.

Homeopathic remedies are derived from plant, mineral, and animal substances, which are soaked in alcohol to extract what are known as the "live" ingredients. This initial solution is then diluted many times, and is vigorously shaken at each dilution to add energy. Impurities are removed and the remaining solution is made into tablets, ointments, powders, or suppositories, or dispensed as drops. Low-dilution remedies are used for acute symptoms (which may be more severe), while high-dilution remedies are used for chronic symptoms (which are often less severe).

Today, homeopathic remedies can be formulated to aid virtually every disorder. However, although the remedies are safe and nonaddictive, the patient's symptoms may briefly worsen. This is known as a "healing crisis" and is usually short-lived. It is actually an excellent indication that the remedy is working well.

It is a common misconception that you can just visit the drugstore, look up your particular complaint on the homeopathic remedy chart, begin taking the remedy, and see marvelous results. If only it were as simple as that! Homeopathic training takes several years, and a lot of knowledge and experience are required before practitioners can determine the correct remedies for complaints other than the most superficial. And, as mentioned earlier, what works for one person may fail to work for another.

Selecting an appropriate remedy is only part of the procedure. The homeopath will also evaluate the patient's reaction to ascertain what, if any, further treatment is necessary. Some women with PCOS have reported that their menstrual cycles normalized within six to nine months after they began taking prescribed homeopathic remedies. However, this information comes from uncontrolled clinical trials; the benefits of homeopathy for women with PCOS have never been properly studied.

Reflexology

Reflexology, an ancient Asian therapy, has only recently been adopted in the Western world. It operates on the proposition that the body is divided into different energy zones, all of which can be exploited in the prevention and treatment of any disorder.

Reflexologists have identified ten energy channels, beginning in the toes and extending to the fingers and the top of the head. Each channel relates to a particular bodily zone and to the organs in that zone. For example, the big toe relates to the head (the brain, sinus area, neck, pituitary gland, eyes, and ears). By applying pressure to the appropriate terminal in the form of a specialized massage, a practitioner can determine which energy pathways are blocked. Minute lumps—like crystalline deposits—detected beneath the skin are broken up by steady pressure. The theory is that the deposits are absorbed into the body's waste-disposal system and removed through sweat or urine, hence restoring the correct energy flow.

Experts in this type of manipulative therapy claim that all the organs of the body are reflected in the feet. They also believe that reflexology aids the removal of waste products and blockages within the energy channels, improving circulation and glandular function. Reflexology is certainly relaxing, and it aids the release of stress. It is also said to be able to help regulate the menstrual cycle.

Many reflexologists prefer to take a full case history before starting treatment. Each session will take up to 45 minutes (the preliminary session may take longer), and you will be treated either sitting in a chair or lying down.

Chapter 7

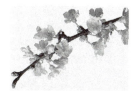

Emotional Support

It is unfortunate that the many physical aspects of PCOS carry with them emotional repercussions. This chapter offers advice and coping techniques to help you overcome these problems.

Your Appearance

Many of the symptoms of PCOS can focus your attention on your appearance. When acne persists beyond young adulthood or when the hair on your head starts to thin in your 20s or 30s, it is doubtless both embarrassing and frustrating. The same applies with weight gain and a darkening or thickening of facial or body hair. To discover on top of other symptoms that you may have difficulty conceiving or that you are classified as infertile can be heartbreaking. It is a sad fact that the symptoms of PCOS can attack a woman's sense of femininity; they can strike a blow at the very heart of who and what she is.

It is no wonder that women with PCOS can lose their confidence. Some even become depressed. All people have doubts about their appearance and have areas of their bodies they don't really like, but if you have PCOS, with its many distressing symptoms, it can seem that nature is conspiring against you. It is challenging to fight a negative self-image, especially when a low mood takes hold, but you only live once, and you owe it to yourself and the people who are close to you to make the most of it.

To give you a kick start in raising your spirits, perhaps you could embark on a course of one of the "stress-busting" herbal remedies described in Chapter 6—preferably under the guidance of a trained herbalist. In addition, you could start a course of one of the other beneficial complementary therapies, with the ultimate aim of reducing your PCOS symptoms. Your improved mood and the feeling that you are helping yourself may provide the boost you need to tackle the emotional effects of the disorder.

Also, consider the following suggestions to help you feel less negative about your body:

◆ Try to stop looking back on the "rosy days" when your body may have been more to your liking. Looking back can only cause further emotional pain, and that's the last thing you need right now. Letting go of the past and focusing on living in the present can give you the strength to tackle the problems you can do something about, such as losing weight or embarking on a course of electrolysis treatments.

◆ Try to accept the things you can't change. PCOS symptoms can be reduced or even eradicated through diet, exercise, stress management, and drug therapy. However, you still may be subject to stubborn symptoms such as thinning hair or acne. If you are doing everything you can to improve your health, resist becoming frustrated if you see little or no change in your symptoms. Keep on trying; it can take many months for the benefits of some treatments to be noticeable. Keep talking to your doctor, too; he or she may be able to offer additional help.

◆ Cheer yourself up by changing your image. A new hairstyle or perhaps a new hair color can work wonders for your confidence, and so can a few changes to your wardrobe. Treat yourself to a facial, an aromatherapy massage, some new makeup. Instead of hiding away, make the most of yourself. A brighter outside can cheer you up on the inside.

♦ Share your worries. Confide in someone close about your concerns about your body image. You will probably find that this person, too, has concerns about herself that you had not even guessed at. If you feel you are deeply affected by the way you look, it may be best to seek the help of a qualified counselor. Your doctor should be able to make a recommendation.

♦ Get regular exercise. Walking, cycling, and swimming are just three examples of activities that raise levels of the "feel-good" endorphins, natural mood-enhancing hormones. Feeling that you have done something good for yourself will help put you in a positive frame of mind.

Boosting Confidence and Self-Esteem

A person who dislikes his or her appearance will automatically have low self-esteem. Whether the problem is with one particular part of the body or several parts, the effect is the same. A woman with PCOS may try to hide a certain part of herself, but at some point she will realize she is not really succeeding, as a result of which she may stop making any effort at all with her appearance. This has a further detrimental effect. Some useful techniques can be employed to counter these negative feelings.

Self-Talk

The way we speak to ourselves has a great bearing on our self-esteem and stress levels. When we stop and take the time to analyze our thoughts, we are often surprised at their negativity—but they must be examined before we can begin to change their destructive pattern. If we drop something, we might think, "I'm really clumsy." If we make an error adding together some numbers, we might think, "I'm useless at math." The same is true if we dislike a particular aspect of our appearance. We might think, "I'm worthless because I'm fat," or, "I'm not feminine, and therefore I'm a freak." A woman with PCOS who's in a relationship might even tell herself she is unworthy of her partner's affection. Such negative self-talk serves only to affirm a woman's deepest fears about herself.

To boost your self-esteem, try to catch yourself every time you have a negative thought about yourself—and instead, counter the thought with one that is positive, for there is sure to be something about your appearance that you can feel happy about. Be completely honest, now. Look at yourself in a full-length mirror and really *see* the positive things. Then maybe you can tell yourself, "I am shapely and have a nice firm bottom," or, "I am voluptuous and have good legs," or, "I have pretty eyes, good hair, and a nice, cuddly figure."

Smile for a While

"All things are cause either for laughter or weeping," wrote the Roman philosopher Seneca. It is true that comedy and tragedy are close bedfellows, for both are reflex actions rooted in the central nervous system and its related hormones.

How we respond to certain stimuli, however, depends on our outlook on life. Letting go of the past and of our fears for the future is "releasing." It allows us to smile more. Laughing at ourselves, in particular, can be more therapeutic than a whole-body massage, it can be more releasing than sex or alcohol, and it invariably makes other people warm up to us. When we laugh, our muscles relax, bleak thoughts lift, and "feel-good" endorphins are released into our bloodstream. As a result, we feel uplifted and brighter!

As we go about our daily routines, we often forget to smile and laugh. Try to make a point of watching funny films and TV comedies, spend time with someone who lifts your spirits, read books that make you smile, and make a determined effort to see the funny side of things. Force yourself to laugh out loud for a few minutes every day. The laughter will quickly become real, and you will feel much better for doing something that felt so silly at first!

List the Positives

When you feel low, take a pen and paper and write down all the good things in your life. These might include having a job you enjoy, a loyal best friend, some great nights out, that old lady who always smiles at the bus stop, the neighbor who often stops for a chat, your dog who gets so excited when you come home.... See what I mean?

Now make a list of all the good things about yourself. Think hard now. There will be a lot more than you might have realized. You may be a good listener, a good cook, have a pleasant singing voice, a good fashion sense, a good sense of direction, a great sense of humor. Don't stop writing until you are sure you've not missed a thing. Once you have finished your list, read it over once again, spending some time appreciating each positive item on the list, and really absorb the pleasure that doing so brings.

Helping Those Close to You Understand

Women with PCOS desperately need to know that the people close to them care. Most of all, they crave the understanding of their nearest and dearest, and they feel upset when they are shown thoughtlessness or impatience.

In attempting to help your loved ones understand the challenges you face with PCOS, be as honest and open as possible. It can be far from easy to speak about the defeminizing nature of the condition, so think first about what you want to say. This section may help you plan what to say.

Communicating Effectively

Before endeavoring to describe your feelings about your disorder, first focus on how you actually feel. It will probably be hard to admit to feeling guilty, frustrated, angry, resentful, useless, and so on, even to yourself, but doing so will help you to come to terms with those feelings and ultimately to let them go. Meanwhile, sharing your feelings with others is an important step toward halting the problems those very feelings can cause.

In your interactions with others, be wary of making assumptions about how they feel about you. For instance, speaking to someone in the following ways is sure to make that person feel he or she is being unfairly judged: "I know you think I'm worrying over nothing, and that makes me really upset"; "I don't believe you could really love someone who's hairy and has zits, and that makes me feel so bad"; "You could try to diet with me. Seeing you eat all that food makes me feel like not bothering." Such comments are likely to be seen as accusations; they may even provoke a quarrel.

Speaking directly about your "emotional issues"—without implying that the other person is contributing to those issues—will help the other person to take your comments more seriously and encourage him or her to be more thoughtful and caring. However, conflicts may still arise on occasion because someone has upset you by doing or saying something hurtful. In such instances, think about the following before you make your reply.

◆ Ensure that you have interpreted the other person's behavior correctly. You may view your mother's bringing you a basket of fruit and vegetables as a criticism of your diet—when in truth it is a goodwill gesture intended to show that she cares. You have a perfect right to interpret the words or actions of others in whatever way you wish, but recognize that your interpretation is not necessarily reality. In fact, it is amazing how often we are wrong in our perceptions of what others think and feel.

◆ Be specific in recalling another person's behavior. Saying "You never understand when I tell you I feel less feminine than I used to" is far more inflammatory than saying "You didn't seem to understand yesterday when I said I don't feel as feminine as I used to."

◆ Make sure that what you are about to say is what you really mean. Statements such as "Everyone thinks you're insensitive" or "We all think you've got an attitude problem" are, besides being inflammatory, incredibly unfair. We have no way of knowing that "everyone" holds the same opinion. The use of the depersonalized "everyone," "we," or "us"—often said in the hope of deflecting the listener's anger—can cause far more hurt and anger than if the criticism is direct and personal.

It is easy to see how others can misunderstand or take offense when we fail to communicate effectively. Still, changing the habits of a lifetime is far from easy. It means analyzing our thoughts before rearranging them into speech. We are rewarded for our efforts when those close to us start to really listen, or when they cease to be annoyed as we carefully explain something they hadn't fully understood.

Dealing with Unfair Comments

Sarcastic and derisive remarks from others can chip away at your confidence. They should not, therefore, pass unchallenged. Standing up for yourself is not always easy, but doing so can have a releasing effect—unlike when you fake indifference or clam up and walk away. In such instances, you may end up feeling hurt, offended, and very resentful. Your most intense feeling, however, will probably be that of anger—at the other person, and at yourself, for allowing yourself to be hurt.

If your partner were to say, "You've put on so much weight...you're not the woman I married," you could calmly answer, "That's a hurtful thing to say. I have put on weight, but weight gain is a symptom of PCOS. I am the same woman, and I still have feelings."

When someone you don't know well makes a comment such as, "I thought you'd have had children by now. Don't you want them?" you could answer with, "I would love to have children, but we don't always get what we want in this life." At this point the person will either be sympathetic, and you will have the chance to reveal more about your problems, if you wish, or the person may probe further, but in a way you find distasteful. He or she may say, for instance, "Aren't you doing everything you can?" It might be tempting to storm away at this point in the conversation, but if you were to do so you would probably be left with the feeling that the other person had gotten the upper hand and that you had allowed that person to hurt you. Saying something to the effect of, "Believe me, there's nothing I don't know about making babies— but actually I don't want to discuss this right now" will make you feel a little better.

Partnerships

It is unfortunate that the distinctive problems experienced by women with PCOS are those that are likely to intrude upon their most important relationship: the one with their partner. For starters, you have to deal with the preconception that intimate relationships should have no secrets. Who wants to tell her partner that she bleaches her facial hair and shaves around her nipples and navel, or that she takes medication to treat acne? Regularly shutting yourself behind a locked door to engage in these routines can leave you feeling guilty.

Women deal with their PCOS in different ways. Most women feel much better when they open up to their partner. Issues they assumed would shock their partner instead generally create a sense of empathy and strengthen the feeling of togetherness. Maybe your partner thought you were being secretive, or that you were having mood swings because you were unhappy. Once a partner has been told the whole truth, and once he has come to grips with his own feelings about the situation, he usually tries to understand.

If your partner really cares about you, he is likely to be concerned about the way you see yourself, about your long-term health, and about how you might cope if you have difficulty conceiving. A small percentage of partners may decide such issues are too much for them to handle and prefer to end the relationship. However, it must be said that this type of person, in the long-term, would probably have proven unsupportive and made you feel worse about yourself. Most likely the relationship would not have lasted forever, even if you hadn't been diagnosed with PCOS.

Initiating a discussion on the subject of a chronic condition such as PCOS can take a lot of courage, but it really is worth it. Try to resist waiting for that "perfect moment" to start talking. Perfect moments never seem to arrive.

If your partner can't seem to understand your problems, the relationship may become a battleground, with each partner feeling resentful and unloved. Unless each person makes an effort to understand the other, the relationship may flounder. It is a fact that you can only truly know what your partner is thinking and feeling when you make time to talk problems through calmly. As a bonus, exchanging perceptions, fears, and needs strengthens your relationship.

If you have tried many times to discuss your problems calmly, and your partner refuses to understand, it does not bode well for the long-term success of the relationship. It's also a fact for women with PCOS that difficult relationships can trigger elevated stress levels and a failure to respond to treatment.

Sex Matters

Whether you are single or involved with a partner, sex is important. Women who are seeking a relationship need to be open to the prospect of sexual intimacy, and that is not always easy for someone with PCOS. Early on in a relationship, it is only human to try to hide parts of the body that are less than perfect, whether it be excess facial or body hair, acne, or areas that you think are too large or lumpy. Before each date you may scrupulously remove every offending hair, apply a thick layer of makeup, and don an outfit that seems to miraculously give you a waistline. It's not easy to keep these habits up week after week, and sooner or later that special person will see a little more of your true self. Once again, we suggest that as soon as the relationship starts to become serious, you resolve to open up about your health problems.

Whether the relationship is fairly new or several years old, women with PCOS can lose interest in sex. It's rarely the act itself that turns them off; rather, they grow to dislike their body so much they can't bear to reveal it. It is only natural to want your partner to think you're attractive, but when you yourself believe that you're anything but attractive, you may recoil at the idea of being seen naked or even seminaked.

The trouble is, if one partner—in this case the woman—appears not to want sex, her partner may conclude that she is falling out of love with him, and the woman may start to doubt the strength of her feelings. If she can admit to not wanting sex because of her appearance, her partner will probably feel some relief. He will probably reassure her that she is worrying unnecessarily and that he still finds her attractive. It is a fact that true love runs far deeper than physical appearance, even if your appearance was part of what attracted your partner to you in the first place. A person is rarely attracted solely by appearance. It also takes personality, shared interests, and like-mindedness to make two people embark on a long-term relationship—at least, on a relationship that stands a fair chance of succeeding.

If you are secure in the core strength of your relationship yet find your sex life has dwindled, talking is undoubtedly the best way to make progress. Tell your partner you feel embarrassed to be seen naked or seminaked, admit to feeling unfeminine, and end by telling him that you still love him. The most likely response will be reassurance that your partner still loves you and still wants to make love with you and that you have no need to feel embarrassed. A night of passion will then be in the cards, which you can prepare for as you wish. Try to make the occasion extra special by lighting candles, by leading your partner to a bubble bath, by wearing that new sexy nightie….

If you can't bring yourself to talk through your issues about sex with your partner, consider seeing a skilled relationship counselor.

The presence of a sympathetic third party may make it easier for you to admit to having problems with your appearance. If you think your situation is too embarrassing to speak about openly with anyone, try joining an e-mail chat room that deals with the subject of PCOS (see Resources). Alternatively, you could see a counselor alone. Ideally you will choose to talk with your partner eventually, and a counselor may be able to give you the support and encouragement you need to take this important step.

Overcoming a Negative Emotional State

Low self-esteem, persistent tiredness, relationship challenges, and anxiety about the future can cause a buildup of emotional stress. We have provided a number of suggestions below that may help you develop a more positive outlook.

Living in the Present

Women with PCOS would be well advised to try to live in the present. A calm and contented *now* is more emotionally nourishing than a mind reeling with the upsets the *future* may hold. In the same way, cherishing the moment is preferable to letting it slip by unappreciated because you are too busy thinking ahead. How many of us look forward to seeing a film, a band, a show, a play—but don't think to enjoy the journey there? How many of us look forward to summer, forgetting to appreciate spring? It is the same with numerous other aspects of our lives.

You may ask, is it possible for someone who dislikes her appearance, who maybe is desperate to have children, to master the art of living in the present? But what is the alternative—to sit brooding on how things used to be, how they might now be, if only...? Wouldn't it be better to read a gripping book, pen a poem, surf the Internet, take a walk, or have a cuddle with that special someone? Admittedly, it is not always easy to lift bleak thoughts, but when you get into the habit of distracting yourself by turning to a pleasurable activity, doing so should eventually become second nature.

Accepting What You Cannot Change

There are many things in life that cannot be changed. Individuals can do nothing about the fact that they are either creative or practical, nearsighted or farsighted, tall or short. Neither can you change the fact that you have PCOS—although you can certainly do many things to improve the situation. Acknowledging what you cannot change—and trying to live with it—is fundamental to stress management, for when you accept things as they are, you say good-bye to a great deal of frustration.

Finding New Interests

As well as offering distraction, taking on a new challenge can be infinitely rewarding and can help you feel more positive about yourself. Consider learning a new language or taking up chess, oil painting, stenciling, playing the piano, line-dancing, tapestry work, glass and china painting, picture framing, jewelry making, gourmet cooking, writing poetry, volunteer work… the list is endless. Or maybe you want to consider an outdoor activity, such as gardening, hiking, golf, sailing, bird-watching, canoeing, or bike riding. Health experts vouch for the fact that spending time outside on a regular basis is a good way to lift a person's mood and promote an overall sense of well-being.

Learning something new can prove very satisfying. Maybe you would like to acquire a few academic qualifications or enroll in a leisure-interest course (where the atmosphere is casual and regular attendance is less important). Studying a subject that is helpful in dealing with PCOS (such as homeopathy, reflexology, aromatherapy, meditation, relaxation, stress management, or assertiveness training) may prove invaluable, too.

What is important is that you choose an interest or course of study that really interests you and that you expect you'll do well at. Failure can be difficult to handle when you are also attempting to come to terms with the effects of a chronic condition or when you're undergoing IVF treatments. Don't forget to congratulate yourself on each small success along the way.

Understanding Chronic Stress

Chronic stress is the state of being constantly "on alert." The physiological changes associated with this state—a fast heart rate, shallow breathing, and muscle tension—persist over a long period, making relaxation very difficult. Chronic stress can lead to nervousness, hypertension (high blood pressure), irritability, and depression.

We have listed below the needs that must be met on a long-term basis in order to avoid suffering from chronic stress.

The Need to Be Understood

Women with PCOS need to feel that the people close to them understand their concerns over their appearance and their worries about the long-term health risks that come with the condition. It is also vitally important to them that family and close friends acknowledge their fears about whether or not they will be able to have children, as well as the myriad emotions that accompany unsuccessful attempts to get pregnant.

When it's obvious that those around you believe you are worrying unnecessarily, you can feel so upset and isolated you begin to shut people out. Recognize that it is not always easy for others to understand how you feel. Taking a deep breath and calmly sharing your feelings is the most important step toward being understood and supported. However, if you have repeatedly tried to help your loved ones understand, and they're still upsetting you, tell them calmly how they are making you feel. Hopefully this will shock them into seeing the situation from your point of view. If not, it would probably be more beneficial to your state of mind to cut yourself off from these people, if possible.

The Need to Be Loved

Feeling unlovable is one of the greatest threats to the emotional well-being of women with PCOS. You may try to tell yourself that appearance isn't everything, yet a concern that your partner finds you unattractive—and so will ultimately end the relationship—may make you subconsciously withdraw your affections. You may even wonder how anyone *could* love you given the way you look. The fear of being unlovable may even have caused you to become irrational and antagonistic.

Before you can be loved by others, you need to love yourself. You need to see yourself as a worthwhile person who posesses qualities that you, as well as others, can respect. Don't let apathy rule. Take the following actions (some of which have been suggested earlier):

- Make a list of your ten best physical attributes.

- Make a list of your ten best character traits.

- Do at least one nice thing (however small) for another person each day, and don't forget to congratulate yourself for doing it.

- Make the very most of your appearance every minute of the day.

- Regularly treat yourself to a therapy that you find uplifting (for example, an aromatherapy session or reflexology massage).

- Indulge frequently in activities that stimulate your mind and create a sense of fulfillment.

The Need to Love

PCOS can cause you to focus wholly on your symptoms, ultimately causing you to withdraw from the people around you. However, loving others and actively attempting to lighten their mood can have a positive impact on your own state of mind. Encouraging your partner to smile will make you smile, too; phoning a friend with relationship problems can cause you to feel useful and good about yourself; showing interest in your lonely neighbor's vegetable garden can hearten you both. Such activities don't require much. You can make someone smile with a few carefully chosen words; a bit of honest flattery will make you feel just as good as the recipient, who will likely be pleased and uplifted by the effort you have made, and who may even want to respond in kind. You have to give before you can hope to receive.

The Need to Be Yourself

The roles many of us play, perhaps unconsciously, often have their origins in early childhood. If the parents of a young woman were always criticizing her for "incompetence," she is likely to grow up with the same attitude about herself. She may develop the habit of hiding instances when she proves to be less than perfect. Only when she moves in with a partner who is far from perfect, a partner who may even be intimidated by her apparent "perfection," will she begin to see that it is all right to be flawed.

There may be several ways in which you hide your real self. Perhaps you dated a person who lived and breathed football. You liked this person a lot, so you read some of the sports pages and feigned an interest that you didn't actually feel. Going through life pretending to be interested in something you don't care a bit about causes untold inner stress. It is far better to be yourself, warts and all. Doing so not only minimizes stress, but also it assures you that the people important to you like you for who you really are.

The Need to Feel Well

Constantly being anxious and miserable can make a woman with PCOS unwell. Fatigue, intermittent pelvic pains, mood swings, and all the other symptoms will only add to that sense. Taking positive steps to tackle the illness should help to counter your lack of well-being. As we've discussed, you can improve matters by eating healthily; getting regular exercise; avoiding exposure to harmful toxins; forging satisfactory relationships with your doctor, family, and friends; learning the art of positive thinking; and trying a few complementary therapies. Whether the benefits are temporary or permanent, the knowledge that you are actively helping yourself creates a sense of achievement and lowers stress levels.

Managing Stress

It is known that a woman who has polycystic ovaries but who lacks any symptoms can develop the syndrome when subjected to a certain amount of stress. For this reason, it is clear that stress is one of the triggering agents of PCOS.

Stress arises not only as a result of what happens to us, but also from our reactions to what happens. Ingrained negative attitudes can actually cause people to see catastrophe in what to others would be normal, everyday events. When a situation is interpreted as a crisis, adrenaline is released into the bloodstream and the body automatically puts itself "on alert." Breathing becomes shallow and fast, the heart rate quickens, blood pressure rises, and the muscles tense—allowing the individual to deal with an emergency more effectively. However, this physiological response can be destructive when it occurs frequently over a long period of time.

Delay Your Reaction

Because living with a chronic condition naturally creates stress in daily life, women with PCOS experience higher levels of stress than nonsufferers. On the flip side, curbing your responses to certain occurrences can greatly reduce the buildup of stress. As a troublesome event unfolds, try to refrain from reacting instantly. Allow yourself time to evaluate the situation—to see it as it really is. Then select a response that doesn't create more stress.

Life-Stress Evaluation

If you take the time to evaluate all the relationships and activities in your everyday life, you are likely to find some that induce a good deal more stress than benefits. At the same time, remember that personal interactions will always produce a certain amount of stress. It is when the stress outweighs the positive gains that you need to consider limiting or ceasing your involvement.

Learning How to Relax

Whether you are struggling to cope with the myriad symptoms of PCOS or undergoing IVF treatment, teaching yourself to relax can make all the difference in your stress levels.

Deep Breathing

In normal breathing, we take oxygen from the atmosphere down into our lungs. When we breathe in, the diaphragm expands and air is pulled into the chest cavity. When we breathe out, we expel carbon dioxide and other waste gases back into the atmosphere. But when we are stressed or upset, we tend to use the rib muscles to expand the chest. We breathe more quickly, sucking in shallowly. Quicker, shallower breathing is good in a crisis, as it allows us to obtain the optimum amount of oxygen in the shortest possible time, providing our bodies with the extra power needed to handle the emergency. However, some people tend to get stuck in chest-breathing mode. Long-term shallow breathing is not only detrimental to our physical and emotional health; it can also lead to hyperventilation, panic attacks, chest pains, dizziness, and gastrointestinal problems.

To test your breathing, ask yourself the following questions:

◆ How fast are you breathing as you read this?

◆ Are you pausing between breaths?

◆ Are you breathing with your chest or your diaphragm?

A Breathing Exercise

Try to perform the following deep-breathing exercise daily:

◆ Make yourself comfortable in a warm room where you know you will be alone for at least a half-hour.

◆ Close your eyes and try to relax.

◆ Gradually slow down your breathing, inhaling and exhaling as evenly as possible.

◆ Place one hand on your chest and the other on your abdomen, just below the rib cage.

◆ As you inhale, allow your abdomen to swell upward. (Your chest should barely move.)

◆ As you exhale, let your abdomen flatten.

Give yourself a few minutes to get into a smooth, easy rhythm. As worries and distractions arise, don't hang on to them. Allow them to float out of your mind, then focus once more on your breathing.

When you feel ready to end the exercise, open your eyes. Allow yourself time to become alert before rolling to one side and getting up. With practice, you will begin breathing with your diaphragm quite naturally—and in times of stress, you should be able to correct your breathing with little effort.

A Relaxation Exercise

Relaxation is a forgotten skill in today's hectic world. We already know that stress, which can give rise to insomnia, hypertension, and depression, is one of the greatest enemies of women with PCOS. It is advisable, therefore, to learn at least one relaxation technique.

The following exercise is perhaps the easiest:

◆ Make yourself comfortable in a place where you will not be disturbed. Listening to restful music may help you to relax.

◆ Begin to slow your breathing, inhaling through your nose for a count of two, allowing the abdomen to expand outward (as explained above).

◆ Now, while ensuring that the abdomen flattens, exhale for a count of four, five, or six.

◆ After a couple of minutes of deep breathing, concentrate on each part of the body in turn, starting with your right arm. Consciously relax each set of muscles, allowing the tension to flow out. Let your right arm feel heavier and heavier as every last bit of tension seeps away. Follow with the muscles of your left arm, then the muscles of your face, your neck, your shoulders, your chest and upper back, your stomach and middle back, your hips and lower back, and finally your legs.

Visualization

After you've consciously relaxed every part of your body, try including visualization in the exercise. As you continue to breathe slowly and evenly, imagine yourself surrounded by a setting that fills you with calm. Perhaps you're in a lush, peaceful countryside, beside a gently trickling stream; or maybe you're on a deserted tropical beach, beneath swaying palm fronds, listening to the sounds of the ocean, thousands of miles from your worries and cares. Let the warm sun, the gentle breeze, the peacefulness of it all wash over you.

The tranquility you feel while doing this visualization can be enhanced by frequently repeating the exercise—once or twice a day is best. With time, you should be able to switch into a calm state of mind whenever you feel stressed.

Meditation

Arguably the oldest natural therapy, meditation is the simplest and most effective form of self-help. The technique can be taught by a teacher, but since meditation is essentially performed alone, it can be learned on your own with equal success.

Meditation involves "letting go" and allowing the mind to roam freely. However, since most of us are used to striving to control our thoughts, letting go is less easy than it sounds.

It may help you to know that people who regularly meditate say they have more energy, require less sleep, are less anxious, and feel far more "alive" than they did before they began meditating. Studies have shown that during meditation the heart rate slows, blood pressure reduces, and the circulation improves, making the hands and feet feel much warmer.

To some people the idea of meditating may seem offbeat. But isn't it worth a try—especially when you can do it for free! Kick off those shoes and make yourself comfortable, ideally in a room where you can be alone for a while. Now follow these simple instructions:

- Close your eyes, relax, and practice the deep-breathing exercise described above.

- Concentrate on your breathing. Try to free your mind of conscious control. Letting your thoughts roam unchecked, try to allow the deeper, more serene part of you to take over. Imagine that your thoughts are a waterfall, and you are simply observing them pass before you. If you find yourself hanging on to any thought or line of thought, just release it by imagining the waterfall resuming its flow.

- If you wish to go further into meditation, concentrate on mentally repeating a mantra—a certain word or phrase. It should be something positive, such as "'Relax," "I feel calm," or "I am a very special person." The aim of mentally repeating a mantra is to plant the positive thought into your subconscious mind. It is a form of self-hypnosis, but you alone control the messages placed there.

- When you are ready to finish, open your eyes and slowly "come back," allowing time to adjust to the outside world before getting to your feet.

In Closing

It should be said that more and more research into the different medications and fertility treatments for PCOS is taking place. While there is often the need for medical intervention in PCOS, there is also a great deal you can do for yourself, for, in the end, the responsibility for your own health lies with you and not with your doctors.

It is best, then, to rope in as many friends and family members as possible to give you support, whether they join you in dieting, sign up with you to become a member of the local gym, or offer encouragement while you are undergoing the emotional rigors of IVF. As we have seen, many of the symptoms of PCOS can be overcome by self-help measures, leaving you free to enjoy your life. On a more personal note, allow yourself to be happy. Do whatever is within reason to achieve that aim. You deserve it, as we all do.

Endnotes

1. I. F. Stein and M. L. Leventhal, "Amenorrhea associated with bilateral polycystic ovaries," *American Journal of Obstetrics and Gynecology*, 1935, vol. 29, pp. 181–91.

2. A. H. Balen, "The pathogenesis of polycystic ovary syndrome: the enigma unravels," *Lancet*, 1999, vol. 354, pp. 966–67.

3. A. H. Balen, G. S. Conway, G. Kaltsas, K. Techatraisak, P. J. Manning, C. West, and H. S. Lisas, "PCOS: the spectrum of the disorder in 1741 patients," *Human Reproduction*, 1995, vol. 10, pp. 2705–12.

4. S. Franks, N. Gharani, D. Waterworth, S. Batty, D. White, R. Williamson, and M. McCarthy, "The genetic basis of polycystic ovary syndrome," *Human Reproduction*, 1997, vol. 12, pp. 2641–48

5. Ibid.

6. D. M. Waterworth, S. T. Bennett, N. Gharani, M. McCarthy, S. Hague, S. Batty, G. S. Conway, D. White, J. A. Todd, S. Franks, and R. Williamson, "Linkage and association of insulin gene VNTR regulatory polymorphism with PCOS," *Lancet*, 1997, vol. 349, pp. 1771–72.

7. A. Dunaif, "Insulin resistance and the polycystic ovary syndrome: mechanisms and implication for pathogenesis," *Endocrine Review*, 1997, vol. 18, pp. 774–800.

8. G. S. Conway, "Insulin resistance and PCOS," *Contemporary Review in Obstetrics and Gynaecology*, 1990, vol. 2, pp. 34–39.

9. P. Acien, F. Quereda, P. Matallin, E. Villarroya, J. A. Lopez-Fernandez, M. Acien, M. Mauri, and R. Alfayate, "Insulin, androgens, and obesity in women with and without PCOS: a heterogenous group of disorders," *Fertility and Sterility*, 1999, vol. 72, pp. 32–40.

10. J. E. Nestler and D. J. Jakubowics, "Decreases in ovarian cytochrome P450c 17 alpha activity and serum free testosterone after reduction

of insulin secretion in polycystic ovary syndrome," *New England Journal of Medicine*, 1996, vol. 335, pp. 617–23.

11. E. M. Velazquez, A. Acosta, and S. G. Mendoza, "Menstrual cyclicity after metformin therapy in PCOS," *Obstetrics and Gynecology*, 1997, vol. 90, pp. 392–95.

12. L. C. Morin-Papunen, R. M. Koivunen, A. Ruokonen, and H. K. Martikainen, "Metformin therapy improves the menstrual pattern with minimal endocrine and metabolic effects in women with PCOS," *Fertility and Sterility*, 1998, vol. 69, pp. 691–96.

13. J. E. Nestler, D. J. Jakubowics, W. S. Evans, and R. Pasquali, "Effects of metformin on spontaneous ovulation an clomiphene-induced ovulation in PCOS," *New England Journal of Medicine*, 1998, vol. 338, pp. 1876–80.

14. A. H. Balen, D. D. M. Braat, C. West, A. Patel, and H. S. Lisas, "Cumulative conception and live birth rates after the treatment of anovulatory infertility: an analysis of the safety and efficacy of ovulation induction in 200 patients," *Human Reproduction*, 1994, vol. 9, pp. 1563–70.

15. A. Abden Gadir, R. S. Mowafi, H. M. I. Alnaser, A. H. Alrashid, O. M. Alonezi, and R. W. Shaw, "Ovarian electrocautery versus human menopausal gonadotrophins and pure follicle-stimulating-hormone therapy in the treatment of patients with PCOS," *Clinical Endocrinology*, 1990, vol. 33, pp. 585–92.

16. R. H. Hall, "The agri-business view of soil and life," *Journal of Holistic Medicine*, 1981, vol. 3, pp. 157–66.

17. F. Goldstein, M. B. Goldman, L. Ryan, and D. W. Cramer, "Relation of female infertility to consumption of caffeinated beverages," *American Journal of Epidemiology*, 1993, vol. 137, pp. 1353–60.

18. K. Kupparanjan, "Effect of ashwagandha on the process of ageing in human volunteers," *Journal of Research in Ayurveda and Sadai*, 1980, pp. 247–58.

Resources

PCOS Support Group

Polycystic Ovarian Syndrome Association (PCOSA)
P.O. Box 3403
Englewood CO 80111
(877) 775-PCOS (775-7267)
E-mail: info@pcosupport.org
Website: www.pcosupport.org
The Polycystic Ovarian Syndrome Association is a national nonprofit organization operated by women with PCOS. The website offers access to chat rooms, e-mail lists, and support groups, as well as links to other online resources.

Verity (UK National Support Group)
The Grayston Centre
28 Charles Square
London N1 6HT
United Kingdom
Website: www.verity-pcos.org.uk

Acupuncture

National Certification Commission for Acupuncture and Oriental Medicine
11 Canal Center Plaza, Suite 300
Alexandria VA 22314
(703) 548-9004   Fax: (703) 548-9079
E-mail: info@nccaom.org
Website: www.nccaom.org

American Academy of Medical Acupuncture
4929 Wilshire Blvd., Suite 428
Los Angeles CA 90010
(323) 937-5514
E-mail: JDOWDEN@prodigy.net
Website: www.medicalacupuncture.org *or* www.acupuncture.com

Aromatherapy

National Association for Holistic Aromatherapy (NAHA)
4509 Interlake Ave. N., #233
Seattle WA 98103-6773
(888) ASK-NAHA (275-6242)
(206) 547-2164   Fax: (206) 547-2680
E-mail: info@naha.org
Website: www.naha.org

Bach Flower Remedies

Bach International Education Program
Nelson Bach USA, Ltd.
100 Research Dr.
Wilmington MA 01887
(800) 334-0843   Fax: (978) 988-0233
Website: www.nelsonbach.com

Depression

Depression and Related Affective Disorders Association (DRADA)
2330 West Joppa Rd., Suite 100
Lutherville MD 21093
(410) 583-2919
E-mail: drada@jhmi.edu
Website: www.drada.org

National Foundation for Depressive Illness, Inc.
P.O. Box 2257
New York NY 10116
(800) 239-1265
Website: www.depression.org

Diabetes

American Diabetes Association
1701 North Beauregard St.
Alexandria VA 22311
(800) DIABETES (800-342-2383)
E-mail: askADA@diabetes.org
Website: www.diabetes.org

Eating Disorders

National Eating Disorders Association (NEDA)
603 Stewart St., Suite 803
Seattle WA 98101-1264
(800) 931-2237
(206) 382-3587   Fax: (206) 829-8501
Website: www.nationaleatingdisorders.org

Eating Disorders Anonymous (EDA)
18233 N. 16th Way
Phoenix AZ 85022
E-mail: info@eatingdisordersanonymous.org
Website: www.eatingdisordersanonymous.org

Electolysis/Electrology

American Electrology Association
P.O. Box 687
Bodega Bay CA 94923
(707) 875-9135
E-mail: infoaea@electrology.com
Website: www.electrology.com

Fertility and Adoption

American Society for Reproductive Medicine (ASRM)
1209 Montgomery Hwy.
Birmingham AL 35216-2809
(205) 978-5000   Fax: (205) 978-5005
Website: www.asrm.org

Holt International Children's Services
P.O. Box 2880
1195 City View
Eugene OR 97402
(541) 687-2202   Fax: (541) 683-6175
E-mail: info@holtinternational.org
Website: www.holtintl.org
Holt International Children's Services specializes in domestic and international adoption and permanency planning for children.

International Council on Infertility Information Dissemination, Inc. (INCIID)
P.O. Box 6836
Arlington VA 22206
(703) 379-9178   Fax: (703) 379-1593
E-mail: INCIIDinfo@inciid.org
Website: www.inciid.org

National Adoption Information Clearinghouse (NAIC)
330 C St., SW
Washington DC 20447
(888) 251-0075
(703) 352-3488   Fax: (703) 385-3206
E-mail: naic@calib.com
Website: www.naic.acf.hhs.gov

Food and Nutrition

American Dietetic Association
120 South Riverside Plaza, Suite 2000
Chicago IL 60606-6995
(800) 877-1600
(312) 899-0040
Website: www.eatright.org

The Price-Pottenger Nutrition Foundation
P.O. Box 2614
La Mesa CA 91943-2614
(619) 462-7600   Fax: (619) 433-3136
E-mail: info@price-pottenger.org
Website: www.price-pottenger.org

The Price-Pottenger Nutrition Foundation, a nonprofit educational organization, is a clearinghouse of information on healthful lifestyles, ecology, sound nutrition, alternative medicine, humane farming, and organic gardening.

Herbal and Nutritional Supplements

ConsumerLab
Website: www.consumerlab.com
A private company founded by a physician and former FDA chemist, ConsumerLab tests nutritional supplements and offers a "seal of approval" if they measure up to certain criteria. Brands that have passed their independent testing are listed on the website.

General Nutrition Centers (GNC)
GNC manufactures and sells vitamin, mineral, and herbal supplements. To locate a store near you, or to order on the Internet, visit the website www.gnc.com.

Shaklee Corporation
Shaklee manufactures and sells nutritional supplements. Its products are available for purchase exclusively from Shaklee Independent Distributors. To locate a distributor near you, visit the website www.shaklee.com or call (800) SHAKLEE.

Homeopathy

National Center for Homeopathy
801 North Fairfax St., Suite 306
Alexandria VA 22314
(703) 548-7790   Fax: (703) 548-7792
E-mail: info@homeopathic.org
Website: www.homeopathic.org

Reflexology

Reflexology Association of America
4012 Rainbow Ste. K-PMB#585
Las Vegas NV 89103-2059
Website: www.reflexology-usa.org

Skin and Hair

The Acne Support Group in Cyberspace
Website: www.voy.com/4529/

Follicle.com
Website: www.follicle.com
A website providing information to those who are experiencing hair loss.

Keratin.com
Website: www.keratin.com
A website discussing hair loss, baldness, alopecia, and excess hair growth.

Further Reading

Best-Boss, Angie. *Living with PCOS*. Omaha, NE: Addicus, 2001.

Dubrow, Terry J. *The Acne Cure*. Emmaus, PA: Rodale Press, 2003.

Gomez, Dr. Joan. *Living with Diabetes*. London: Sheldon Press, 1998. (Visit www.sheldonpress.com.)

Hammerly, Milton, and Cheryl Kimball. *What to Do When the Doctor Says It's PCOS*. Rockport, MA: Fair Winds Press, 2003.

Harris, Colette, with Dr. Adam Carey. *PCOS: A Woman's Guide to Dealing with Polycystic Ovary Syndrome*. New York: HarperCollins (Thorsons), 2000.

Harris, Colette, with Theresa Francis-Cheung. *The PCOS Diet Book: How You Can Use the Nutritional Approach to Deal with Polycystic Ovary Syndrome*. New York: HarperCollins (Thorsons), 2002.

Holford, Patrick. *The Optimum Nutrition Bible*. Berkeley, CA: Crossing Press, 1999.

Holford, Patrick, and Kate Neil. *Balance Hormones Naturally*. Berkeley, CA: Crossing Press, 1999.

Holmes, Elizabeth. *The Natural Way: Acne*. London: HarperCollins, 2001.

Liew, Lana, with Linda Ojeda. *The Natural Estrogen Diet and Recipe Book* (2nd ed.). Alameda, CA: Hunter House Publishers, 2003.

Index

gestational diabetes, 22
ginseng, Indian, 92
ginseng, Siberian, 93
Glucophage, 21–22, 34, 41, 44
glucose-tolerance test, 28–29, 41
goldenseal, 81
gonadotrophin releasing hormone
    (GnRH), 16, 44
gonadotrophin therapy, 42–44
grains (diet), 56–57
green tea, 52

H

hair, excessive. *See* hirsutism
hair loss (alopecia), 2, 80
hemp oil, 8, 81
herbal remedies, 90–94; ashwa-
    gandha (Indian ginseng), 92;
    echinacea, 93; *Rhodiola rosea,* 92;
    sarsaparilla, 81, 93; Siberian gin-
    seng, 93; St. John's wort, 93–94;
    vitex agnus-castus, 91–92; white
    peony, 93
heredity and PCOS, 13–15
high blood pressure, 14, 24
hirsutism, 2, 5; and bleaching, 79;
    and depilatory creams, 78; and
    electrolysis, 77–78; family history
    of, 14; and laser hair removal,
    80; medications, 31, 32–33; and
    photothermolysis, 80; and shav-
    ing, 79; and waxing, 78–79
holistic medicine, 87. *See also* com-
    plementary medicine
homeopathy, 83, 94–95
human chorionic gonadotrophin
    (hCG), 18
hyperandrogenism, 20, 31
hyperglycemia, 21
hyperinsulinemia, 21
hypoglycemia, 21

hysterosalpingogram (HSG), 40

I

in vitro fertilization (IVF), 44–46;
    success rate of, 45–46
infertility, 5–6, 10; family history of,
    14
insulin, 20, 21–22, 28–29, 50
insulin resistance, 13, 21, 31; medi-
    cations for, 34–36
intercourse, timing of, 39–40
intercytoplasmic sperm injection, 45
interests, importance of, 108
intrauterine device (IUD), 32

J

jasmine (aromatherapy), 86–87
joint pain, 3

L

laparoscopic ovarian diathermy,
    42–43
laparoscopy, 40
laser hair removal, 80
laughter, importance of, 100–101
lavender, 86, 94
legumes, 55–56
lemon balm, 94
Leventhal, Michael, 3
luteal phase, 17, 18
luteinizing hormone (LH), 16, 19, 28

M

meal plans, 58–60
medications, antibiotics, 8, 30;
    clomiphene citrate (Clomid), 36,
    41–42; combined oral contra-
    ceptive pill (COCP), 31; cypro-
    terone acetate, 31; Dianette, 31;
    drospirenone, 31; finasteride, 33;

ONCE A MONTH: Understanding and Treating PMS ... 6th Ed.
by Katharina Dalton, M.D., with Wendy Holton

This book introduced the world to premenstrual syndrome, proving that it is a real—and treatable—condition. Originally written in 1978, this sixth edition introduces a whole new generation to PMS. One-third of the material is new, from research on how PMS affects learning to the PMS/menopause connection. Dalton also addresses the whole range of treatments, including progesterone therapy, and self-care methods such as eating something starchy every three hours.

320 pages : 68 illus. : Paperback $15.95

ANDROGEN DISORDERS IN WOMEN: The Most Neglected Hormone Problem *by Theresa Cheung*

Androgen disorders are imbalances of the "male hormones" (androgens) that cause excessive facial and body hair, unusual hair loss, acne, weight gain, menstrual dysfunction, ovarian cysts, and an increased risk of heart disease and diabetes. Many women are embarrassed to discuss these symptoms with doctors. This book will help them understand and manage the problem. It includes case histories, interviews, descriptions of conventional and alternative treatments, and a section on prevention and self-help.

208 pages : 7 illus. : Paperback $13.95

ANEMIA IN WOMEN: Self-Help and Treatment *by Joan Gomez, M.D.*

The symptoms of anemia—shortness of breath, fatigue, headaches, and lapses of concentration—can easily be attributed to the stress of modern life. But undiagnosed anemia can lead to infertility, premature delivery, fainting, and mental confusion. Joan Gomez discusses why women develop anemia more than men, the two main types of anemia, their treatment, and self-help options. Whether a woman is a teenager, a mother, or a grandmother, she should be educated on this silent disease.

176 pages : Paperback $12.95

THYROID PROBLEMS IN WOMEN AND CHILDREN: Self-Help and Treatment *by Joan Gomez, M.D.*

More than half of all thyroid disorders remain undiagnosed because the symptoms are attributed to other diseases. Yet thyroid problems are 90 percent curable and relatively easy to treat. This book helps readers understand the health impact of thyroid disorders and the treatment options. Special chapters cover pregnant women, infants and children, adolescents, and women over 50 and discuss vitamins, the role of iodine, and the role of stress in thyroid problems.

208 pages : Paperback $12.95

All prices subject to change